CITIZENS AT THE CE

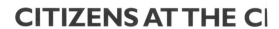

Deliberative participation
healthcare decisions

Celia Davies, Margaret Wetherell and
Elizabeth Barnett

First published in Great Britain in October 2006 by

The Policy Press
University of Bristol
Fourth Floor
Beacon House
Queen's Road
Bristol BS8 1QU
UK

Tel +44 (0)117 331 4054
Fax +44 (0)117 331 4093
e-mail tpp-info@bristol.ac.uk
www.policypress.org.uk

British Library Cataloguing in Publication Data
A catalogue record for this book is available from the British Library.

Library of Congress Cataloging-in-Publication Data
A catalog record for this book has been requested.

ISBN-10 1 86134 802 9 paperback
ISBN-13 978 1 86134 802 9 paperback
ISBN-10 1 86134 803 7 hardcover
ISBN-13 978 1 86134 803 6 hardcover

Celia Davies is currently Director of the Research for Patient Benefit Programme at the National Institute for Health Research. **Margaret Wetherell** is Professor of Social Psychology at The Open University. **Elizabeth Barnett** is ex-Research Fellow in the Faculty of Health and Social Care at The Open University, now retraining in psychotherapy.

Cover design by Qube Design Associates, Bristol.
Front cover: photograph kindly supplied by Robert Harding World Imagery.
Printed and bound in Great Britain by Hobbs the Printers, Southampton.

Contents

List of figures and boxes

Figures

Boxes

Acknowledgements

This book represents the culmination of a long collaborative journey. Consequently, our debts of gratitude are many. First must come our co-workers in research, foremost of whom was Sarah Seymour-Smith who organised the collection and transcription of an extraordinary quantity of video data and who played a key role in the first analysis of this material for the evaluation study. Next is Helen Sheldon, then of the College of Health, who, despite significant setbacks, interviewed the individual members of the Citizens Council and created and analysed that dataset. Our sound and camera crew of Vince Wells, Colin Bright and Bill Eustace supported us with understanding and creativity. We must also thank Shirley Lyman and Chris Nichols for patient hours of transcription and quantitative analysis. The Open University provided us with some time and space to reflect beyond the final report stage; without this, the very idea of a book would have been impossible.

The National Health Service (NHS) Research & Development (R&D) Methodology Programme provided funding for the evaluation project on which this work was based. We would like to acknowledge this, and also to record our particular thanks to Richard Lilford and Judith Harris for their generosity and support at a moment of near disaster. The views and opinions expressed in this book, however, are those of the authors and do not necessarily reflect those of the Methodology Programme or of any other parties involved.

The National Institute for Health and Clinical Excellence (as it is now) was the organisation whose innovative initiative we were evaluating. Despite the sometimes delicate nature of our task and their own ever-growing workload, all the key organisational players gave us of their time and their insights, kept us 'in the loop', and allowed us to be part of the furniture of their working lives. Our greatest thanks go to Ela Pathak-Sen, the project manager of the Citizens Council, who moved with grace and helpfulness across boundaries of organisation, contracted agency, individual citizens, and an ever-curious evaluation team. Without her support and friendship our research would have been impoverished. Her senior colleagues – Mike Rawlins, Andrew Dillon, Andrea Sutcliffe and Peter Littlejohns – welcomed us into the rarefied world of strategic level thinking and planning. Similarly we are grateful to the staff of Vision 21 in general, and Ruth Turner and

Simon Danzsuk in particular, for their cooperation in sharing the inner workings of recruitment and facilitation with us.

Above all, however, we must give tribute to the members of the Citizens Council themselves. After a nervous start, they treated us as fellow pilgrims in an ongoing search for understanding, and brought us into their company with honesty, generosity and humour. Without their cooperation there would simply have been no story for us to tell. We hope they will feel that we have made good use of all their efforts.

Finally we want to thank June Ayres, Penny Wilkinson and Sarah Pelosi of The Open University and Alison Shaw and her colleagues at The Policy Press for their patience, hard work and creativity in taking our text and turning it into a book. As authors, we must take responsibility for judgements and errors in the text. The finished product, however, is more than our words; it is the labour, generosity and understanding of all who have shared our journey.

A note on terminology

We have taken certain decisions with regard to terminology in writing this book that we think it would be helpful for the reader to have set out clearly at the outset.

While still using the acronym 'NICE', today this organisation is the National Institute for Health and Clinical Excellence. When it was originally set up, and throughout the period of our study, it was the National Institute for Clinical Excellence. It was not until April 2005 that it joined with the erstwhile Health Development Agency and acquired a longer name. It was decided to retain the original acronym (NICE) since this was how it was best known to the public. In-house staff tend to refer to it as 'the Institute'. We have therefore chosen to refer to it either as 'NICE' or as 'the Institute'.

Although the names of all the members of the Citizens Council are in the public domain, and have been since NICE first posted them on its website, we have nevertheless sought to preserve confidentiality within the body of the text by the use of fictitious individual names. Each member chose their own pseudonym. In doing this we have been able to quote individuals and demonstrate important aspects of deliberative behaviour without identifying individuals.

Within NICE the Citizens Council is always written without an apostrophe – as is the Institute's Partners Council. This is grammatically correct as it is a proper noun, and has well-known precedents, such as Friends House in London. Despite this, some commentators have wished to introduce an apostrophe. We have chosen to follow the Institute's own practice, and refer to the Citizens Council unapostrophised.

Introduction

Governments today are asking citizens to come forward to participate
in political decision making, not just locally but on a national stage, to
debate some of the most complex, and the hardest decisions of our
time – about science policy, for example, health, environmental issues,
world poverty and global resource use. But how feasible is such a
demand? We are often told that citizens are more sophisticated and
reflective than ever before. They are better informed, they weigh
options and make myriad personal and family choices. Yet they
have become less loyal to leaders and more critical of governments.
Their lives are busy and diverse; many have become individualistic,
inward-looking and disengaged. Fewer are turning out to vote in
national and local elections. Both severe economic and social
inequality, and privilege and social advantage can turn out to be
sources of political disconnection. Even if people are willing to
participate in a direct way, is there a corpus of knowledge,
imagination and understanding capable of creating the kind of
political space in which citizens feel comfortable and can make a
contribution? Assuming questions such as these can be resolved
satisfactorily, there is still the issue of where direct citizen participation
fits in relation to the existing political institutions and the
accountability structures that they entail. Citizen participation is
undoubtedly in fashion right across western democratic states. But
that does not mean that there are not hard questions to be asked of
it.

Calls for more citizen participation have arisen against a
background of change. New social movements have done much to
force the pace. Greens, feminists, minority ethnic groups and people
with disabilities, to name but a few, have provided powerful critiques
of policy directions. Some of these groups now find themselves at
the policy table alongside industrial and trades union interest groups
in a more complex stakeholder dialogue where governments are
anxious to portray themselves as more flexible and responsive.
Engaging directly with the public is a theme that attracts political
parties of all hues as they attempt, in this context, to shed old
ideologies, reposition themselves beyond left and right, and grapple
with the complexities of just what kinds of legislative interventions
are imperative and acceptable. In the new forms of governance that
have been emerging, governments have increasingly relinquished

roles as direct service providers, instead becoming standard-setters and monitors. They are turning to focus groups, citizens' juries, roadshows and listening exercises, in the hope of gaining more of a sense of what it is that citizens want in a world where the old certainties of political ideology are no longer in play.

Different interpretations both of 'the citizen' and of 'participation' are involved in this move towards more 'modern' governance (Newman, 2001, 2005). Frequently citizens are seen not as citizens at all, but as 'consumers'. Here the role of government is to ensure that there are competing providers of goods and services among which consumers choose, and it is the sum of individual choices, plus market research on the part of the providers, which shapes what is available. To address a 'citizen' is to imagine a more active actor, integrated in a polity and participating collectively in decisions about what is to be done. In practice, participatory initiatives frequently address a more specific, hyphenated citizen – the citizen-resident, with an interest in the site for a new local facility, or the citizen-service user, with views on how services could be changed to better fit their lives and the experience they have had. These are important distinctions, not least because it is easier for hyphenated citizens to know who they are, and what experience they can call on as relevant to the situation at hand. Democratic innovations initiated by local government often turn out to be of this sort: addressing the citizen-resident as someone likely to be fairly directly affected by a decision outcome.

In contrast, when people are called on to participate as citizens by central government, the issues they are asked to debate are likely to have less immediacy and the link between citizen identity and experience is likely to be more tenuous. Citizens and their hosts may need to make an imaginative leap to enter the world of the other if real dialogue is to take place. This adds an important further dimension to the troubles that arise in any citizen participation arena – the challenges, for example, of motivating citizens and generating commitment to the task, of handling complex information and the recurrent questions of representation and representativeness.

Just how much is known already about all of this? In one sense the answer is 'a lot'. Local government has long had its consultative machinery, using advisory committees and public meetings and in recent years has brought in a range of other innovations in democratic practice in trying to reach out and bring in the people it serves. Parent and pupil participation in the running of schools, patient participation in the running of doctors' surgeries and hospitals, and service user groups in fields such as learning difficulty and mental health have all come strongly to the fore. Arnstein's five-rung ladder of involvement, first developed in the 1960s as a challenge to town planning authorities in the US and a call for partnership with citizens, is one device that figures prominently in many case studies and evaluations (Arnstein, 1969). Running from no involvement at all and information provision and public relations on the first rungs, to joint decision making and then complete service user control at the top, it can be used to assess and evaluate participation of different kinds and levels. It is applicable both in the context of involving specific service user groups and in the context of public or citizen participation more broadly. Few initiatives today are to be found located on the very bottom rungs of the ladder, but equally there are few examples where responsibility is shared or where power has been handed over to service users themselves. Studies that utilise Arnstein's ladder often remain small-scale and localised – what they share is a challenging and a critical commentary, demonstrating that pre-existing power relations all too easily remain intact. Arraying and assessing techniques and toolkits for participation, however, is a growing activity (Mullen, 1999). Some international coordination is occurring, for example, through the International Association for Public Participation (www.iap2.org).

When we ask, however, what is known at national level about forms of involvement in the machinery of central government, the picture is more shadowy. Diverse initiatives can be identified. Most visible, perhaps, are the actions of governments in taking contentious topics out to the people – not just issuing a formal consultation document and waiting for written replies, but publicising the issue, setting up focus groups and holding meetings around the country attended by the relevant minister. Creating a public debate or perhaps a form of citizens' jury to come to a verdict on what might be done and why has become more common. Alongside this are the actions taken by those charged with the responsibility of carrying out a public enquiry to get involved face-to-face with those with an interest, and to find ways of soliciting public opinion on the matters on which they must pronounce. One recent high profile example is the way that those charged with enquiring into the high profile deaths of babies at Bristol Royal Infirmary rethought their procedures and the setting of their work, in order to encourage participation from parents and the public (Secretary of State for Health, 2001). Another example comes from the Committee on Radioactive Waste Management, one of whose initial principles was to take full account of public and stakeholder views (Blowers,

2005), and who indeed caused controversy and came under fire, as some thought, for going too far and ignoring expertise (see, for example, *The Guardian*, 31 October 2005). Accompanying all of this, there has been a now long-running effort to broaden recruitment to public bodies and to address their lack of public accountability. Some paint these diverse moves on a broad canvas of reconfigured and networked governance, and as part of a complex and contradictory project, remaking people, publics and politics (Newman, 2005). As yet, however, sustained, micro-level empirical attention to the realities and consequences of these different forms of participation is rare.

In among all this searching for practical ways forward, one theoretical perspective has become particularly significant. People are increasingly called on not simply to react as individuals or to represent particular constituencies, but to work together to digest relevant information, and to engage in discussion with others whose social positions differ markedly from their own. In a word, the aim is that they should *deliberate*.

What is deliberation? The term is much used and is often used loosely. Locating it firmly in the political science debates in which it has its origins, however, it becomes a well-specified theoretical idea, with assumptions about what citizen participation entails and what putative advantages it can bring. Deliberation understood in this context is a vision of a group of highly diverse and strongly motivated citizens, given resources and support. They are assigned a question and provided with access to the knowledge underlying different viewpoints. They are encouraged, often by a facilitation team, to reflect on this and to explore how far they, as a group, are able to reconcile conflicting positions on complex issues.

Deliberation is attractive to different people for different reasons. Political philosophers have been intrigued by the theoretical possibilities of deliberation as a form of action which is potentially not oriented to power and interests. Within political science more generally, the topic signals and opens up debate about deliberative democracy as a putative new political form, transcending some of the limits of more conventional, liberal, representative democracy. There is also a growing interest in innovative institutional design – in developing and assessing ways in which a vision might translate into practice.

Another and rather broader source of appeal lies with the positioning of deliberation firmly in the territory of the social, and its valorising of the emergent character of social action. Deliberation is very importantly about what people bring to the table, but it is also about what they can achieve in interaction with each other. It holds out the possibility of new understandings that none would have reached singly – and for the social integration and sense of community that such an experience is likely to encourage. Reasserting the value of the social at a point where there is so much emphasis on individualism, and where rational choice theories are in the ascendant, can be appealing to scholars in social policy, sociology and social psychology.

Particularly intriguing is the way in which the idea of deliberation has entered the discourse of contemporary politics. The popular work of sociologist Anthony Giddens (1998: Chapter 3) in the UK captured this in his call for 'democratising democracy' and his emphasis on deliberation as heralding a chance for a more 'generative politics', going beyond what many have come to see as tired ideological attachments. The associated notion of 'third way' politics may have fallen out of favour, but a stream of publications on experience of citizens' juries, with a message which we will consider in some detail in the body of this book, that 'people can do this', has been brought to the fore by UK think-tanks, thus finding its way by a different route into ministerial policy thinking.

But is this utopian? Is it simply a fantasy on the part of socialist radicals who have been looking for a new home in recent decades? To any social theorist, the requirements of deliberation are going to look strenuous to say the least. Deliberation requires an assembly of citizens from across the social spectrum; people who would not encounter each other in the course of normal daily life need to work together. They will call on norms of sociability, politeness, courtesy and consideration for others. They will also need to accommodate different vocabularies and styles of interaction if they are to share experience and ponder on the implications of its distinctiveness. Alongside this they will need to learn, engaging with unfamiliar ideas and variable formats of information presentation; some, perhaps most, will also worry about their own abilities to cope. Will they even come forward to take part? And if they do, will they actually stay the course? Is it feasible that all viewpoints will be both articulated and heard in such an arena?

There are both optimistic and pessimistic responses to such questions. Cooke and Kothari (2001) fall into the latter camp. Introducing a collection of essays in the field of development studies, they offer a stark provocation with their concept of the 'new tyranny' of participation. Bringing local citizens into direct participation for sustainable development in projects in India, South Asia and elsewhere has become the orthodoxy, they say, and almost all would concede that top-down, externally imposed and expert-oriented initiatives have severe limitations. But, in taking this route, they argue, an ostensibly radical discourse of citizen participation ends up reinstating the very power relations it aims to overturn. There are *sotto voce* conversations among both participants and practitioners about what goes wrong, and there is difficulty and embarrassment about putting questions and criticisms firmly onto the table. Close to the other extreme is the optimistic writing of those working in the West who advocate citizens' juries and other participatory initiatives, emphasising citizen capacity in face of elitist doubt. (Some of this work will be considered more fully in Chapter Two of this book.) Fung and Olin Wright, bringing together accounts of a participatory local budget in Brazil, of initiatives in devolved development powers in India, and two governance-sharing projects in the US, argue that these are examples of "empowered participatory governance". They are practical forms that "elicit the energy and influence of ordinary people", and empowered participatory governance is a concept that "presses the values of participation, deliberation and empowerment to the apparent limits of prudence and feasibility" (Fung and Olin Wright, 2003b: 5). Their aim is to instate a notion of 'real utopias', drawing out new theorising from these case studies – theorising shaped by a political vision of institutions free from oppression, and seeking to give this practical expression in principles of design. Empowered participatory initiatives must be carefully distinguished from those, regardless of the intentions of designers, which limit and constrain. The reference to *grounded* citizens' juries in recent work on a smaller scale in the UK signals a similar point, arguing that the issues discussed must be grounded in the concerns of a local community, deliberation must be meaningful to participants, and the results must be shown to have affected the circumstances of local people's lives (Kashefi and Mort, 2004). Does this mean that today's emphasis on participation initiatives that are government-led will inevitably turn out to be mere 'technologies of legitimation'? Introducing this pessimistic-sounding concept, Harrison and Mort (1998) suggest that citizen participation is unlikely to determine or shape policy in a direct way, but they leave open the possibility that it has the capacity to inform and educate and also, importantly, to improve accountability.

This book is the outcome of a sustained effort to examine closely a high profile initiative at the heart of government policy concerns. Working with citizen participation inside the institutions of regulatory government at national level, the authors have traced the creation of the Citizens Council in the health service standard-setting body the National Institute for Clinical Excellence (NICE) from its announcement as a brief line in the government's NHS Plan in 2000 to its implementation, and we have followed, over a period of two years, events at the first four Council meetings. Time spent observing the host organisation as it designed the Council and worked with an outside agency to shape the meetings, repeat interviews with the citizen members themselves, and, above all, video-recording and transcribing all the main sessions of the Council and many of its subgroups gave access to a level of detail and inside insight not previously achieved in research on citizen participation.

There are several important features of this. First, we are able to ask what happens when you come to deliberation as a researcher committed to building from the bottom up, carrying out a fine-grained and detailed ethnography of the interactions that occur. Informing the detailed case study analysis is the question: just what kind of a *social practice* is citizen participation and what are its consequences? How, for example, does citizen participation unfold *in situ* and how does it become discursively established? Second, we have been able to pay close attention to context. How, in the absence of some of the novel design features of government institutions specified by Fung and Olin Wright, do the micro-, meso- and macro-level influences interrelate to shape and reshape possibilities for deliberation? How too are we to reconcile, if reconciliation is necessary, the assessments of participants and those we ourselves make as observers?

Third, choosing deliberation as the central point of reference, and focusing in depth on interactional data as we do, has consequences for what the book is not, as well as for what it is. Readers with some knowledge of NICE will be aware of the intense debates, taken up in Parliament and in the media at the time of the creation of NICE, over whether the Institute, developing guidelines on the effectiveness and efficiency of drugs and clinical procedures, served to mask political choices about rationing the services that the NHS should offer. They will be mindful of the way in which interests, including patient group interests, can be mobilised as particular drugs come under scrutiny, to contest the randomised controlled trial evidence and ask for a different assessment of the balance between evidence and experience in the final decision. In the period since completion of our data collection, a wider public has begun to become increasingly aware of the way in which NICE guidance opens up fundamental political debates about the potential for setting rules about restricting treatments, not on the grounds solely of clinical decisions of need in individual cases, but in terms of criteria that may or may not have the support of public opinion: according priority to younger patients for example, or denying treatments to those whose past lifestyle decisions make the prognosis bleak. Awareness that values necessarily entered decisions on clinical effectiveness and cost-effectiveness was a factor that stimulated interest in the creation of a Citizens Council as a way of keeping in touch with public values. For all these reasons, readers might expect to find 'content' in this book – in the shape of a direct examination of values held by citizens, and values changed as a result of membership of the Council, and of the reasoning underpinning recommendations that NICE take a particular stance on hard choices and controversial issues. Such an approach can be traced most clearly in the recommendation from the Council to NICE, discussed in Part II of this book, that denial of treatment on grounds of age (a 'fair innings argument') was unacceptable. But this is a book that is fundamentally about process rather than about substance. It does not develop the kind of insights that can be drawn from a research design that measures values at time 1, administers an intervention and measures again at time 2 (see, for example, Dolan et al, 1999). Instead its focus is on the character of the intervention itself – on citizen deliberation. We will argue that citizens do not bring already formulated values to a deliberative arena in any clear way at all. And we will demonstrate the power of discourse analysis to bring new kinds of understanding to the processes of citizen participation itself, regardless of the specific context in which that participation occurs.

Deliberation, as portrayed in the literature of political science, thus remains the key axis on which the book turns, but, by the end, the deliberative ideal that it constructs (teased out and explored in Chapter Two) has come into question. The shackles of current deliberation theory need to be loosened, we argue, if citizens are to find an expertise space in which to operate. This is particularly so when deliberation moves from the local to the national, and from the concrete to the more abstract. And the place of citizen deliberation in the further embedding and renewal of democracy is by no means yet securely established.

Outline of the book

Part I explores the wider context in which the detailed case study that forms the heart of this book is set. Citizen participation has become a major preoccupation of governments in many western countries as they seek to find new ways to integrate those whom they rule, and gain greater legitimacy for their actions. Chapter One examines the way that this entered into the policy discourses of the Labour Party in the UK, tracing how citizen participation meshed with the project of renewing the Party in the long years of opposition in the 1980s and 1990s, and then infused policy and practice when the Party came to power in 1997. Nearly 10 years on, there have been a number of experiments with face-to-face citizen assemblies, designed to discuss strategic policy issues. We examine examples of several of these, highlighting the way old and new discourses intertwine, and underlining chequered histories. Policies around both patient and public participation in the health sector are also traced, providing a context for the case study that is to come. Britain's NHS may have been the jewel in the crown of the mid-20th-century welfare state, but by the late 1990s it was being concluded that its ways of working and seemingly sluggish performance stood in need of strong infusions of direct participation by discerning and critical citizens. We show how the arrival of NICE, and the idea of a Citizens Council that would work alongside patient and other stakeholder groups in this still new organisation, fitted into this.

Deliberation, and the circumstances in which citizens might become deliberators, is the subject of Chapter Two. The aim, carving a pathway through the dense, complex and long-standing debates among specialists in political science and political philosophy, is to tease out just what kinds of social practices this notion of deliberation entails. Some of those most deeply engaged in the theoretical debates have themselves taken on the practical task of creating new institutions and structure – the notion of a deliberation day is a striking example (Fishkin, 1995). Our argument is that theory stands in need of new and rather different understandings. These, we claim, can be derived largely from social psychology, but there is also a need to call on those who can bring a critical and analytical edge to the contexts of deliberation and to policy analysis, if this field is to advance. We outline an approach from theories of social practice and from discourse analysis that is then followed through in the rest of the book.

The four chapters of Part II focus on the Citizens Council of NICE as a case study in citizen participation. The Council met four times for periods of two and more days during our two-year study period, and these meetings were video-recorded and transcribed. Interviews were conducted with the 30 Citizens Council members at the outset and again towards the end of the study. An in-house

Institute steering group met regularly through this period, planning the sessions and monitoring the results, with a member of the research team in attendance. We were thus able to observe how key groups within the Institute, its Board and Partners Council reacted, sometimes by questioning both procedures and results. (For more on research methods and data, see Appendices 1 and 5.)

This rich set of data sources has given us an opportunity to visit and revisit transcripts of interaction in a way, we would argue, that has not been open to previous researchers. The results reveal a story of citizens keen to participate, yet struggling to come to terms with the question set and to find ways of being with each other, their hosts and facilitators which drew on their past experience in what was a highly unfamiliar situation. There was much experimentation and adaptation across the set of meetings as the worlds of hosts and Council members, over time, began to come into closer alignment. Even on a minimalist definition, however, the amount of deliberation remained small. The power of a social practice approach and of discourse analysis in tracking the sense-making activities of participants, and the often covert way in which power relations become instated in an emerging community of practice, is demonstrated in Chapters Four, Five and especially Six.

The opportunity to come alongside those with the responsibility to design and implement the Citizens Council initiative, both those in the host organisation and those in the facilitation team with whom they contracted to support the citizens and run the meetings, gave us an opportunity to extend the analysis significantly. NICE had to interpret what to them was a novel task of setting up a Citizens Council, fleshing out what was at first merely a couple of lines in a health policy document. A new, still controversial form of government regulator, the Institute also had to position the Citizens Council in relation to government sponsors and immediate stakeholders in and around it. We bring into the analysis some of the discursive work which this involved (see Chapters Three and Seven). 'Context' emerges from this as more complex and nuanced, less fixed than in other accounts.

What ultimately was the impact of the initiative? 'Do you want to improve the NHS?' had been the lead question in the recruitment literature for the Citizens Council. People came forward in very substantial numbers in response (see Chapter Three). The vast majority of those selected not only stayed the course, but reported to the research team that their experience had made them keen to find ways of continuing to be participating citizens. And yet, as we shall see, the questions that they were asked did not relate in any straightforward way to improving the NHS, and the answers given in the reports of the meetings caused considerable bemusement and disquiet within the organisation and among stakeholders.

Part III examines the implications of the case study findings, moving away from a success/failure calculus to try to spell out what can be learned about creating an expertise space for citizens, and confronting in a more subtle way than hitherto the questions of citizen capacity and power that arise. We do this in two ways. Chapter Eight engages critically with deliberation theory as it has developed in political science, asking what happens when this is viewed from rather different disciplinary eyes and with the benefit of detailed ethnographic data. We argue for an expanded understanding of deliberation as practice and a move away from the particular forms of political science theorising that have so far dominated debates. Chapter Nine turns to practical politics. It develops a series of seven messages addressed to those who seek to design deliberative initiatives, embed them in existing institutional structures, and in the process perhaps transform understandings of just what 21st-century democracy might mean. Both chapters address what we see as the over-expansion and under-analysis of citizen deliberation, and in doing so pose different sets of challenges for the future.

Readers can choose various pathways through this work. Practitioners charged with the task of setting up a citizen forum, for example, may wish to start at Chapter Three and use the case study as a trigger for their own thinking about the context in which they are placed, the opportunities it offers, and the different ways in which an event might be structured to help bring a group of citizens onto the unfamiliar terrain of policy. This is not the 'how to' book that they may be seeking – but the reflection it generates, and the messages contained in Chapter Nine, may usefully supplement manuals offering specific techniques. Students, by contrast, may wish to focus on the first two chapters in order to gain a quick insight and entry to the conceptual area of participation and deliberation – perhaps skipping to the reframing of this in Chapter Eight, before mining the case study chapters for points of particular interest or debate.

Policy makers have little time to read full-length academic books. They might find the conclusions to the chapters helpful, or they might well want to turn to the bullet points of the executive summary in the research report that preceded this book (Davies et al, 2005). Those who advise them, however, those who straddle the worlds of policy and academia, the academics in the different disciplines who have separately engaged with this issue, and the deliberation theorists are the readers we most hope to attract. There is a debate to be had, as the concluding chapter makes plain, about deliberation and about the death and the potential rebirth of collective action in 21st-century politics, which can be glimpsed through the findings reported here. Perhaps this book will stimulate others to see further.

Part I
Context

ONE

The rise and rise of participation

> And our third term? Well the good work we have begun must continue, but there is also an opportunity for people to enjoy the public realm as never before: for people to have more of those enriching shared experiences that make life worth living, that nurture a common sense of humanity and that remind us that our shared citizenship goes a lot deeper than just the right to vote. (Jowell, 2005: 11)

The idea of direct participation of the public in the business of collectively governing their lives has been a vision and an aspiration that has fascinated politicians, political theorists and political commentators down the centuries. In contemporary times it can be seen, for example, in the intense interest across western democracies associated with Robert Putnam's work on the collapse of civic engagement in the US and its potential for revival (Putnam, 2000), and in talk of a need for greater social solidarity and cohesion. It can be seen too in the flurry of work in political science on 'deliberative democracy' which will be discussed in detail in Chapter Two. The hope expressed in the opening quotation by Tessa Jowell, at the time Secretary of State for Culture, Media and Sport in the UK government, also reflects this. For her, the vision of citizen participation calls up the possibility that people might influence in a very direct way the environment and services that are available to them – not just by reading the newspapers or watching television, but by having a say in hard decisions about issues of resource allocation and policy direction. She wants a new focus on what the 'public realm' could and should be: creating a collective solidarity and combating what she calls a 'poverty of aspiration' to engage with politics. At the particular moment of her writing – in April 2005, as New Labour prepared for a third term of office – this was the *refreshing* of an ideal, building on a theme of democratic renewal that had already been threaded through reformed structures of governance under the banner of modernisation. In visionary political writings such as these, troubling questions about the conditions under which 'enriching shared experiences' for citizens could be produced in the public realm, quite reasonably perhaps, can be set aside. The empirical conditions that might make participatory practice possible, the sites in which it might occur, and the nature of the constraints that might surround it, however, are at the heart of this book.

This chapter offers an introduction to debates about democratic renewal and direct citizen participation as they are being played out in Britain in the early years of the 21st century. The first section takes up notions of a more active citizenry, paying particular attention to the way in which these have been developed by New Labour in its project of modernising governance and seen by commentators and critics. It highlights the crucial link between hopes for participation, the reform of the state and the project of democracy. Political ideas, however, need to take a specific form drawing on existing institutions and organisational practices as well as seeking to instate the new. The next section gives a glimpse of the fate of some recent participatory practices as they have been tried at national level, and the sense of disappointment and betrayal that they have generated. Local level cases are more frequent and can be more positive, but it is only recently that authors have begun to classify and categorise and to tease out contradictions. In the third section, the chapter considers how these themes are playing out in the sphere of health. This is a particularly interesting case for two reasons. First, there is the legacy of separation between the NHS and local government, and the history of attempts to infuse localism, service user voices and consumer responsiveness into what from the outset has been a sharply hierarchical system of accountabilities is a particularly fraught one. Second, the NHS is important, also, as the setting for the detailed case study which is presented in Part II of the book and which raises a number of key questions in this field. Will citizens come forward to address complex issues and face hard choices in public policy? Are they prepared and able to take on the complex scientific and technical issues which underpin such decisions? If the answers to both of these questions are 'yes', what are the features of a good participatory design? What too are the outcomes, and who is to weigh the costs and the benefits? The chapter closes by underlining some of the unresolved issues that surround exercises in citizen participation. In doing so, it starts a move from the specificities of one time and one place, to the broader issues of theory and practice that will be tackled next.

Participation and the policy discourses of New Labour

A Labour government came to power in May 1997 on a tide of excitement and anticipation after 18 years of Conservative rule. At the Labour Party conference later that year, Tony Blair was to recall the drive home from Buckingham Palace. The people watching the journey on television who then poured out of doorways to wave and clap, he felt, were "yearning for change in their country at a time when they could see that we had the guts to modernise and change our Party" (quoted in Fairclough, 2000: 115). Rather more discretely and quietly, many of the civil servants, having experienced the rigours of competition, market testing and outsourcing, were also keen for a different era of relations between the state and its citizens to begin. They faced a new and very inexperienced government, but it was one with seemingly more respect than its predecessors for the public sphere and what could and should be achieved there. Euphoria apart, the incoming government had to steer a delicate course. It had won a clear victory on the ticket of New Labour – distancing itself on the one hand from the market-oriented, neoliberal ideas deeply entrenched under the Conservatives, and on the other from the socialist traditions of old Labour. 'Both and ...' was the theme. Strict economic competitiveness would be squared with social cohesion; there would be efficiency and entrepreneurial bite together with a new and strong emphasis on social justice, and the public and private sectors were now to work together in a productive partnership.

The late 1990s had produced a ferment of ideas for an alternative government programme as those on the Left reviewed the mantra of the market, the depth of economic and social inequalities, the rolling back of the state and the seeming passivity of the public in the face of this. Labour's Commission on Social Justice, set up in 1992 and based at the left-of-centre think-tank the Institute for Public Policy Research (IPPR), had taken forward the crucial idea of a social investment state (CSJ, 1994). While in opposition, politicians had listened to the ideas circulating in academia and the media. Two slim volumes by the editor of *The Observer* caught the mood in the run-up to the election – serving as a rallying cry that linked the parlous state of the nation with the parlous state of the state (Hutton, 1995, 1997). Associated with this was much commentary on the potential of a 'third way'. Back in 1989, the BBC Reith Lectures by sociologist Anthony Giddens under the title of 'The runaway world' had begun to characterise for a general audience the depth of economic and social change that any radical government needed to acknowledge. There were the forces of globalisation on the one hand – and there was a less deferential public, more suspicious of authority, more concerned with lifestyle politics on the other (see also Giddens, 1991). The mid-1990s saw the start of what was to be a series of short accessible texts on the third way – the reconstitution of politics in this changed environment (Giddens, 1994, 1998, 2000).

Twin ideas of enhanced citizen participation and a new project for the state were at the very heart of this analysis. In a world where "traditions have to explain themselves" (Giddens, 1994: 5), the basis for social cohesion or solidarity has to be built anew. Government, Giddens' argument had implied, must neither seek to provide for and control the citizen (as in old Labour), nor to abdicate to the market (as in the New Right). Eleven positive roles were listed (Giddens, 1998: 47-8). Among these was the creation of a revived public sphere where government must engage and generate active trust among a differentiated citizenry. In this context, a radical politics is a politics that deliberately courts participation and dialogue. It is not so much about rights and the representation of interests: "it creates forms of social interchange which can contribute substantively, perhaps even decisively, to the reconstitution of social solidarity" (Giddens, 1994: 113).

These ideas found a strong echo with the incoming Labour government. Alongside measures to strengthen the economy, people were exhorted to come forward to contribute to debates about the future direction of the country and the shape of reformed public services, which could be capable of being more responsive to changing need. All this signalled nothing less than a new revitalised and refreshed kind of democracy. 'New politics for a new century' was the subtitle of a pamphlet published by Prime Minister Tony Blair in 1998. "The democratic impulse needs to be strengthened", he argued, "by finding new ways to enable citizens to share in decision-making that affects them". He explained:

> For too long a false antithesis has been claimed between 'representative' and 'direct' democracy. The truth is that in a mature society representatives will make better decisions if they take full account of popular opinion and encourage public debate on the big decisions affecting people's lives....

It was not just a matter of a more mature society:

> The demand for more democratic self-governance is fed by better educated citizens and the free-flow of information provided by new technology and the media. We must meet this demand by devolving power and making government more open and responsive ... diverse democratic debate is a laboratory for ideas about how we should meet social needs. (Blair, 1998: 15, 17)

This is not to say that there is a perfect match between academic theory and political practice. Labour in opposition and in power drew on and made a selective reading of a range of related ideas as they circulated through political networks. Think-tanks such as Demos and the IPPR were important. There were other sources too – ideas emerging from the US, for example, and from Europe (Fairclough, 2000). Nor is it to say that a new political discourse comes tidily packaged, is coherent and perfectly formed; this was as untrue of Blairism as it was of Thatcherism before it. Distance from the daily events, and a tendency to retrospective glossing both by participants and commentators, will serve to 'overtidy' what in practice are more hesitant, messy and contested forms of discourse. The concept of the 'third way' in particular came in for considerable criticism for its contradictions and ambivalence and its lack of a 'big idea' (see, for example, Cutler and Waine, 2000; Powell, 2000; Lister, 2001). Close readings of political speeches and official documents show how some formulations were dropped, while others proved more durable (Fairclough, 2000). Nor again should it be assumed that a new discourse represents a clean break from the past. Labour's early economic policy and caution on public spending, and its retention of an internal market in health, albeit much softened, are examples of this. Finally, there is the question of 'events'. One example here is the unanticipated ferocity that surrounded professional self-regulation in face of the high profile case of baby deaths in surgery at the Bristol Royal Infirmary (Kennedy Report, 2001). Mixed messages about the importance of professionals for the new public service agenda ensued (Davies, 2003). Undoubtedly, however, and in terms of the broad-brush account here, more direct and immediate citizen participation was one of the key and continuing themes in New Labour discourse after 1997. If this was so, how did it work out in plans for new forms of institutional practice?

With an immediate focus on restructuring arrangements for both central and local government, health, education, social welfare, the criminal justice system and so on, 'modernisation' of public services came to serve as a better lead idea than the third way (Newman, 2001). There was no gainsaying the truth of tired and dilapidated schools and hospitals. They needed investment (which would not be forthcoming in any major way until the second term). But, building on Conservative constructions of the public as discerning consumers rather than the grateful citizen inheritors of the 1940s' welfare state, New Labour – at this point at any rate – wanted citizens not to opt out of public services but to become actively engaged in quality improvement and renewal.

At first, organisational and managerial changes predominated. This was true of the initial health White Paper, for example, notwithstanding that a key principle was "to rebuild public confidence in the NHS as a public service accountable to patients, open to the public and shaped by their views" (DH, 1997: para 2.4). It was true also of plans for social care. Once again, a language of user and particularly carer empowerment was visible in the policy document, but the main modernisation of services was to be secured through managerial measures rather than democratic ones (DH, 1998). The new discourse of citizen participation emerged altogether more directly in relation to local government. Figures for average turnout in local elections in the European Union showed Britain at the bottom of the table. The government wanted to turn this around.

'In touch with the people' was the subheading for a 1998 White Paper (DETR, 1998). It argued for a thoroughgoing change of both structures and culture. Councils, as Minister John Prescott explained at the outset, needed to break free from old-fashioned attitudes that planned and ran services for local people, and to be prepared instead to listen, lead and build up their local communities. New mechanisms to combat paternalism and inward-lookingness by directly elected mayors, cabinets, more frequent elections and the use of referendums on local issues were some of the changes proposed at this stage. There would now be a statutory duty to consult local people about plans and to involve them in how services could be improved. The document explained that:

> ... modern councils fit for the 21st century ... are built on a culture of openness and ready accountability. They have clear and effective political leadership, to catch and retain local people's interest and ensure local accountability. Public participation in debate and decision making is valued, with strategies in place to inform and engage local opinion. (DETR, 1998: para 1.2)

Innovations in democratic practice at local level had in practice been attracting attention for some while (Stewart, 1996). The policy document acknowledged this. The Census of local authorities in England that it had sponsored early in 1998 found citizen participation being encouraged, not only through traditional public meetings and consumer surveys, but also through standing citizen forums and panels, as well as through more interactive consultative and deliberative events. On average, each local authority used nine different forms of such activity during the Census year. It seemed that there was "a momentum behind the participation agenda that extends beyond any individual method". The political colour of the authority had little effect and the researchers commented that:

> [T]he rapid take-up of new forms of participation suggests a latent disposition within local government for much greater public involvement and an enthusiasm for developing new opportunities. (Lowndes et al, 2001a: 210)

What then of citizen participation at the centre? Government thinking and its plans and progress reports have become more accessible to the public – at least to those able to use the Internet and with the time and inclination to browse. On the No. 10 website it became possible, for example, to take a virtual tour of Downing Street, to email the Prime Minister, and to trace speeches and documents. Action to deliver on the citizen participation discourse can be identified in at least four areas. First, and most visibly, there have been a series of initiatives, mainly with short-life funding attached, where the government has attempted among other goals, to galvanise greater citizen participation. Examples here include the whole field of activity focused on tackling multiple deprivation in local areas, the neighbourhood renewal strategy that started in the newly formed Social Exclusion Unit. There was a Community Empowerment Fund, designed to resource more effective mechanisms for direct involvement of local people. There have been specific attempts to bring particular voices into the policy process. One such attempt was the 'Better Government for Older People', a programme launched in 1998, and led from the Cabinet Office, supporting 28 projects across the country, each setting its own objectives for joined-up service improvement for older people based on direct consultation with older people themselves (Hayden and Boaz, 2000).

Second, a spotlight was being turned on how government departments and agencies themselves might work more openly and inclusively. A code of good practice to be used by government departments when consulting on policy directions emerged in 1998 and was later updated (Cabinet Office, 2004). Departments were enjoined to appoint in-house consumer champions. The question of appointments to non-departmental bodies came under scrutiny. 'Quangos: Opening the doors' (Cabinet Office, 1998a) aimed to build public confidence through making quangos more open, capable of being understood and attractive to potential appointees. The Committee on Standards in Public Life insisted on advertisements of posts and interviews. Yet it seemed that the 'old boy network' was not totally swept away (Davies, 2001), and a MORI poll showed just how distrustful the public still were on this topic (Elgood and Mountford, 2000). As Labour started its second term, new targets for diversity in public body membership were set (Cabinet Office, 2002).

Two additional moves are discernible. One was the clear shift towards integrating stakeholder groups, including consumer and service user groups, quite directly into the policy development process. The development of the NHS Plan as an exemplar of this is examined later in this chapter. The other was a move to try to make central government more 'in touch', most obviously through the use of focus groups, but also, as the next section will show, through forms of direct engagement such as the 'Big Conversation'.

How can all this be summed up? A new participative discourse was now enmeshed with and developing out of the older one concerned with 'consumers'. Managerial ideas were also now jostling with notions of greater accountability to relevant publics. But there was also a local/central dimension. Late in 1999, the Public Administration Committee was taking evidence for what was to become a report under the title *Innovations in citizen participation in government* (House of Commons Select Committee on Public Administration, 2001a). At local level, the repertoire of innovations was considerable. But the role of public participation in central government, declared Professor John Stewart, was frankly a puzzle (House of Commons Select Committee on Public Administration, 1999). Were central departments trying more imaginative ways of consultation? The answer appeared to be 'yes' – but developments were fragmented and sporadic, and seemingly good ideas pursued with apparent enthusiasm could all too easily find themselves the target of criticism from sceptics, idealists or both. Stewart was right to question whether there was any strategic direction.

The next section gives a flavour of arrangements put in train in recent years to involve people not so much as users or consumers of a specific service but as citizens. It then begins to ask not so much the question government is so fond of posing, 'what works?', as 'what contradictions are revealed by the present kinds of practices that are instated under the banner of citizen participation?'

Participation in practice

As Labour moved into a second and then a third term of office, the call for citizen participation did not go away. If anything, it built up more of a head of steam. Agencies external to government continued to press for the strengthening and deepening of democratic innovations, with friends now in high places. The IPPR in the mid-1990s, for example, had been a particularly strong advocate of the idea that complex and controversial topics could be tackled with the use of citizens' juries (Stewart et al, 1994; Coote and Lenaghan, 1997). Some key advocates found themselves in advisory roles in government, although an IPPR review in 2002, as we shall see below, kept up the pressure for change in Whitehall (Clarke, 2002). Closer to home for the government were two reports. The Public Administration Committee renewed its call for action in its report on democratic innovation (House of Commons Select Committee on Public Administration, 2001a) following a dramatic drop to a 59% turnout in the 2001 Election (House of Commons Select Committee on Public Administration, 2001b). A little earlier, the House of Lords Select Committee on Science and Technology was also advocating more dialogue between the experts and the public (2000).

The boxes set out below detail some specific ways in which the government tried to give substance to the notion of participation and to create new kinds of participatory practice at national level. None proved to be without difficulty. At its launch, the People's Panel (Box 1.1) was hailed as "proof positive that we are a listening government" by the then Minister for Public Service (Cabinet Office, 1998b). Commentators were more critical. The objectives were never clear and it tended to be used as "an *ad hoc* market research tool for departments and agencies seeking a quick turnaround in fieldwork" (Clarke, 2002: 41). Nor was it the 'world first' claimed in the publicity statement. Evaluators had identified attrition and the 'conditioning' of remaining panellists as undermining its value. The Select Committee echoed the criticisms, calling for an altogether more imaginative use of the Panel (House of Commons Select Committee on Public Administration, 2001a: para 70; see also Pratchett, 1999; Smith,

2005:33). All this, not surprisingly, meant that the press could present it as an expensive gimmick.

Box 1.1: The People's Panel

The People's Panel was established in 1998 from within the Cabinet Office, with the help of market research organisation MORI and the School of Public Policy at the University of Birmingham. It was hoped that it would provide a group who could be asked about their experience of a variety of public services. It was to enable views to be followed over time and to help government to understand reactions to its services as a whole. A total of 5,000 members of the public were recruited so as to be representative of the population of the UK as regards age, gender, region and a range of other demographic indicators. Reserves were also recruited and an additional 830 minority ethnic members were included to boost the sample and facilitate comparison. In principle, the Panel was to be available to all government departments and other publicly funded bodies. Five waves of research covered themes including the levels of service people expect and complaints handling. Transport, local democracy, housing, gas safety and out-of-hours services were among the more specific topics. Some departments tried to use the Panel to recruit focus groups; one, for example, on issues of concern to women. The Panel was wound up in January 2002. Its total cost had been £869,000.

The same fate was suffered by The Big Conversation. As Box 1.2 indicates, however, it ran onto the rocks in a rather different way. Its name proved to be very close to that of an independent political conversation website, where apparently much more critical comments, including comments about the Prime Minister, were being posted. The press had a field day, judging the initiative as just so much more government spin.

Box 1.2: The Big Conversation with the electorate

Launched in November 2003, to coincide with the Queen's Speech on the opening of Parliament and with a lengthy document on future policy, this was presented by the Prime Minister as the biggest consultation ever with voters. A website was set up to enable people to email their views directly, so that the government might keep in touch with thinking in the country. It was to be a step towards delivering on the pledge to keep in touch with the people. By the following spring the government

---

found itself embroiled in controversy. Emails, perhaps intended for the government's site, were in practice being addressed to a pre-existing and similarly named website. The owner of the latter accused the government of censoring the kind of criticism that was emerging. The Big Conversation was dropped; Internet visitors found themselves being redirected to the Labour Party's website.

The issue over whether to promote genetically modified (GM) crops proved equally challenging. All the indicators were that there was much public suspicion of such a move, although the basis for this view was unclear, and on the part of the industry hopes for commercial exploitation were high. The government agreed to a public debate on a scale not previously experienced in the UK, although there were precedents, not least in Holland's 'Great Debate' (see Chapter Two, Box 2.2).

Box 1.3: 'GM Nation?' A public debate on GM crops

Prompted by an advisory body, and aware of the controversies being generated by the topic, in the summer of 2003 the Department for the Environment, Food and Rural Affairs (DEFRA) appointed an independent steering committee to oversee a process of public participation. 'GM Nation?' included a number of dimensions. Eight initial workshops of 18-20 participants from different age groups and parts of the country debated the issues for consultation and materials to be used. There was also a ninth workshop for people actively involved in the issue. Around 675 open meetings were held debating the materials including a specially produced film. Ten focus groups stratified by age and socioeconomic status provided a comparison group. The total cost was in excess of £650,000. DEFRA commissioned a review of the relevant science and a cost–benefit study to set alongside the public debate. An independent evaluation was also carried out (Horlick-Jones et al, 2004, cited in Smith, 2005: 116, n 65).

The evaluators criticised 'GM Nation' among other things for inadequate resourcing, failure to bring those previously uninvolved into the debate and a lack of space for genuine deliberation. Looking a little later, Wilsdon and Willis (2004) point to timing as a particular issue – it was established much too late in the process to influence the directions of research. Also the visions of key players (they single out the commercial company Monsanto) were not opened up for scrutiny in an effective way. In their view it was never made fully clear just why the initiative was occurring. Following the work of Stirling (2005), they highlight three potential reasons for taking such initiatives. Reasons can be normative (that it is the right thing to do); they can be instrumental (that initiators need to anticipate likely reactions in order to present policies in the best light); or they can be substantive (that more robust solutions and better outcomes will emerge). If the reasons are substantive, and the authors of this book argue that they should be, then there is a case for the government to see the views that emerge not as 'another ingredient in the pot' but as directly shaping the ultimate decision. Not all would agree. At local government level there is a fair amount of consensus, whatever the results that emerge from citizen participation events, that accountability and hence the final decision should be in the hands of elected representatives (see, for example, Lowndes et al, 2001a: 213; Newman, 2001). We return to this important point in Chapter Two and again later in the book.

The need for clarity about objectives was becoming a more insistent theme. The IPPR review had been particularly scathing. It suggested that Whitehall "appears unsure and often unwilling to move beyond the traditional consultation approach", and that it was hence "underperforming on the public involvement agenda"(Clarke, 2002: iii). It is worth underlining as Smith (2005: 35) does, however, a point made by the GM evaluators. This experiment would have been quite unthinkable a decade earlier.

Two years on from the GM debate, the citizen participation issue at national level was still very much on the table. It was clear, what with the events around GM foods, the BSE scandal before it, the questions that were now arising over developments in genetics in relation to human reproduction, and the related theme of stem cell research, that the public was losing confidence in both the scientists and government. The potential of nanotechnology was gaining more and more press coverage. Was there learning to be had from the handling of GM? Could public participation be introduced in a better way? In the summer of 2005, Nanojury UK was launched (see Box 1.4). Developed independently by a group with experience of the DIY jury model (Wakeford, 2002), it gave more scope for citizens to set the agenda and to have direct control over their report, and seemed set to avoid some of the problems that had been experienced in the GM debate. At the time of writing, however, it was unclear what reception the findings would have and where they would figure in the decision processes of government.

Box 1.4: Nanojury UK

During the summer of 2005 a partnership made up of a science lab (University of Cambridge), a campaign group (Greenpeace UK) and a group of action researchers (based at the Policy Ethics and Life Sciences (PEALS) Research Centre, University of Newcastle) designed and sponsored a process that was then facilitated by PEALS. Twenty people from a wide range of backgrounds took part. A two-way model was used, first allowing the citizens to set an agenda of their own (youth crime and exclusion in their area). Only after the jury had worked together on a local issue on which they were passionate were they introduced to the second stage of the process, focusing on nanotechnology. Several jurors stopped turning up at this point. Those remaining (between 12 and 16 attended) were introduced to the subject by three dramas about new technologies, enacted by the facilitators. The jury then met over 10 evening sessions to evaluate evidence on the role that nanotechnologies might play in the future. The witnesses to be heard by the jury were chosen jointly by the scientists and an oversight group. Working according to the established DIY jury model (Wakeford, 2002; PEALS, 2003) the report was to be in the form of recommendations, drafted by the jurors themselves after rolling small group discussion. The jurors also created several mini-dramas portraying positive and negative future scenarios for nanotechnology. The aim was to feed the report to a government group charged with coordinating views on this topic. *The Guardian* newspaper was also part of the initiative, undertaking concurrently to run a forum both online and in the newspaper to enable others to comment.

Two reports became available in 2005, in their different ways seeking to bring together the learning that could be distilled from the various initiatives – locally and centrally. The POWER Inquiry was set up as an independent commission with funding from the Joseph Rowntree Trust to explore how democracy might be increased and deepened in Britain. Working to a brief set by the Inquiry, Smith (2005) presented almost 60 democratic innovations from around the world, describing and classifying them and exploring what generalisations could be gleaned. His conclusions lent support to imaginative and innovative measures. At the same time, he warned that culture change was often required, that no technique was perfect, that combinations were often indicated and that nothing came cheap. Work carried out under the auspices of the think-tank Demos, focusing on science and technology, was more critical. It concluded that few democratic initiatives in the field of science either involved citizens early enough or allowed their questions to shape the process. Without this, citizen participation initiatives would fail to address issues of public concern – questions such as:

> Why this technology? Why not another? Who needs it? Who is controlling it? Who benefits from it? Can they be trusted? What will it mean for me and my family? Will it improve the environment? What will it mean for people in the developing world?

The challenge, they insisted:

> ... is to force some of these questions back on to the negotiating table, and to do so at a point where they are still able to influence the trajectories of scientific and technological development. (Wilsdon and Willis, 2004: 28-9)

On the topic of involvement and participation, it seems, fine words can all too easily backfire. In a climate of raised expectations, activities that, viewed from the government side of the fence, go a considerable distance beyond previous practice can be fiercely contested. The next section takes a closer look at the trajectory of developments in what has come to be known as patient and public involvement (later, engagement) in the field of health. In doing so, it provides a more detailed example of the hesitancies and confusions that have surrounded the rise of citizen participation. It also serves to set the scene for the detailed case study in Part II.

And in the field of health?

The notion of engaging in any direct way with the public was not part of the mindset of policy makers when the NHS was established in 1948. Voters had given their strong endorsement to the idea of a national health service and to state welfare provision. A unified and hierarchical NHS structure that looked upwards to the Ministry for guidance was the result. It reflected a belief, on the one hand, in the expertise of the medical profession and the self-evident value of its services, and, on the other, on the potential of a system of public administration to deliver. It sidestepped local authority control and accountability to elected representatives – anathema to the doctors. The roles of the local dignitaries who were the lay appointees on hospital management committees and regional boards were not clearly defined, but in no sense were they representatives of service users or citizens (Klein, 2001: 59).

The first break with this settlement with the public came with the creation of Community Health Councils (CHCs) in 1974, designed to provide a voice in the NHS from the local community. CHCs combined voluntary association members (often with a specific interest in mental health, for example, or children's services) with local authority appointees and those from NHS regions. There was a right to information, and a right to be consulted over hospital closures and major changes to local services. But CHCs were outside the new system of management introduced at the same time and designed to create a stronger consensus between the clinicians and administrators. Over the following years, there were moments of high profile media attention, as CHCs carried out their own surveys of local services or came together nationally to build a picture of what was going wrong. There was much local variation in activity, however, and CHCs could be dominated by casework and individual complaints handling. In the main, their odd mix of service user and citizen interests was accommodated by the NHS, rather than representing a radical transformation of it (Webster, 1998; Klein, 2001).

A second break with top-down control emerged in the Thatcher years. There were two strands here. First, accompanying the belief in the importance of the market came an emphasis on understanding *the customer*. For all its focus on strong management, the report from Roy (later Sir Roy) Griffiths, at the time deputy chairman and managing director of the Sainsbury supermarket chain, pointedly observed that businesses, unlike the NHS, "have a keen sense of how well they are looking after their customers" (Griffiths, 1983: 10). The government donned the mantle of customer care in its official statements and ministerial speeches, and hospitals and general practices began to publicise performance figures and carry out satisfaction surveys. Second, almost as a by-product of the emphasis on business principles and competition, a stronger citizen strand emerged. With a new purchaser–provider split, health authorities were now contracting for services on behalf of a local community. *Local voices*

(NHSME, 1992) enjoined them to give local people an opportunity for influence. Some authorities engaged the public in priority-setting exercises through surveys, workshops, health panels, discussion groups and citizens' juries. Others brought local councils and voluntary organisations, for example, into stakeholder discussions. Still others, however, building on expertise in epidemiology and public health, interpreted the task as calling for in-house expertise in quantitative techniques of community profiling, needs assessment and rapid appraisal (McIver, 1998: 9). The twin moves of the markets era thus opened up new NHS participatory practices, in some ways paralleling the democratic innovations of the local authorities.

The influences that prompted participatory developments – in health and in local government too – were by no means all driven by formal politics. Pressure from below in the shape of organised service user groups is important. The increases in confidence and voice that were apparent in this period can be traced further back (see, for example, Klein, 2001: 89). One dramatic example of demands on government for participation came from those with learning disabilities, under the much-used slogan 'nothing about us without us'. Baggott et al (2005) map the growth of health consumer groups, linking this with the decline of deference, the rise of issue politics, and cross-cutting influences, from feminism, for example. Such groups now, they suggest, are seeking directly to change discourse and practice, and with their alliances, networks and coalitions are finding a place at the policy table (cf Hogg, 1999; Wood, 2000).

There was another important factor. The challenge of finding resources in the face of ever-rising expectations and increasingly costly new treatments was also emerging onto the political scene, not just in the UK but much more widely (Coulter and Ham, 2000). If things could no longer be left implicit, was there a rational and technical fix to be had or was it a matter of widening participation and engaging in political argument? For government and the medical profession, the former was attractive. Under a growing banner of evidence-based care, a new health technology assessment research programme got under way in 1993 and a centre was set up to generate systematic reviews on the efficacy of clinical treatments. Guidelines on clinical treatments began to emerge from various quarters; health economists found a voice – a single metric for the quality of a life year (QALY), for example, appeared to hold out hope of rational rationing decisions. By the late 1990s, however, the volatile politics of all this was all too apparent (Ham and Robert,

2003). The controversies provoked by the Oregon Plan (a list of treatments made available under the US Medicaid scheme) were well known; closer to home the 'Child B' case, where a trust had denied expensive treatment for a child dying of cancer, had been headline news. The other route was to bring the public in to the business of making hard decisions. Citizens' juries were tried by a number of local authorities. NHS trusts now also took up the idea. Some years later, drawing together experience across five countries, Ham and Robert (2003: 15) saw the dichotomy between the two approaches as a false one. What was needed was a way of amalgamating the two – an 'informed democratic consensus model'.

By the time that New Labour forged the programme that was to bring it into power in 1997, it was clear that both patient and public involvement had already risen significantly up the agenda for the NHS under previous administrations. Something more decisive needed to be done about participation. Under the NHS Plan (DH, 2000), patients were to be directly empowered through rights of access to records and information; there were new duties on trusts to collect patient feedback and penalties for those who did not act on the results of the now annual patients surveys. CHCs and a creaking complaints system were to be swept away. The new organisational arrangements, enshrined in legislation in 2001, introduced a Patient Advice and Liaison Service, a new independent complaints service, together with Patient (later Patient and Public) Involvement Forums. For the first time, elected local authority members were given a direct role in assessing local NHS services through what were to become overview and scrutiny committees.

Equally important, however, was an acknowledgement at this point that government *nationally* had to work in a new way. In health (and in other areas too), the intention was that the government took a step back from control of service delivery to setting standards and priorities. It now saw itself as performance managing against set criteria and only intervening where organisations were failing to meet these. But standard setting and monitoring had to mean "more inclusive local and national structures" (DH, 2000: para 6.8). Already there were new faces in Whitehall. Service users had participated in the setting of standards for various care groups and conditions in the production of the new National Service Frameworks. The production of the NHS Plan had itself mirrored this inclusion. Patient groups were represented on the Modernisation Action Teams that preceded it and were the direct signatories to the Plan.

A reading of policy documents of this period, both in the health field and beyond, however, reveals a fusion and perhaps confusion of ideas. There is a failure, for example, to distinguish clearly between the participation of people as consumers/service users and that of people as citizens. Older notions of 'consultation' and 'involvement', and newer and more active ones of 'participation' and 'engagement', are often run together. A wealth of critical commentary and research has emerged in health and in other fields. Some of the issues that it identifies are practicalities; how to defend the necessary resources of money and time against direct spending on services is one example; just how interested citizens can be assumed to be, how to recruit them and how to deal with objections about 'unrepresentativeness' is another. Other issues centre on independence and the potential for capture, raising questions about the motives of those who invite citizens to participate. The tenor of both activist and academic commentary is often sceptical and even cynical – asking whether this is something that is 'cosmetic' only, 'lip service' or 'tokenism'. We have already seen some of the challenges on this front in the science policy field. Peck (1998) has argued that the key need in practical policy terms is to face quite directly the issues of integrity, ambiguity and duplicity that arise. Harrison and Mort (1998), taking a more sociological view, suggest that both public consultation and user involvement can be seen as 'technologies of legitimation' in what has become an increasingly pluralistic policy arena. Lowndes et al (2001a and b) offer a particularly vivid and nuanced account of how local citizens' views can be significantly misaligned with those from within the local authorities. One recent article underlines the limits of what local government, working within statute, can deliver (Williams, 2004). Another stresses the importance of starting where citizens are, acknowledging their negative experience with local government, and working to overcome this (Rowe and Devaney, 2003).

Facing these ambiguities, citizens, as the material in this book will show, cast around for just what is expected of them and draw on diverse ways of positioning themselves in relation to participatory initiatives. Finding a position from which to speak, as citizen rather than service user, in a national rather than a local arena, in relation to a more abstract issue of policy direction and strategy, and in relation to a group of others drawn from a diversity of social backgrounds, is a particularly unfamiliar and challenging task. Both explicit and implicit framings in the policy framework and event design are likely to have an impact.

Policy development around participative practices in health has not been smooth sailing. Recently, the government has tried to force the pace, with guidance on implementation and good practice (DH, 2003; Vivian, 2004), but its own commissioned studies show up some of the conflicts and mixed motives that beset the field (Farrell, 2004). A reallocation of powers and responsibilities at the centre had to follow when the still very new Commission for Patient and Public Involvement in Health proved to be a casualty of a review and cull of the number of arm's length bodies (DH, 2004).

The Citizens Council of NICE represents a high profile initiative set within this overall context. NICE was set up as one of the new standard-setting and regulatory agencies after 1997, charged with the responsibility of developing national guidance on drugs and other interventions for the NHS. It was already acknowledging the importance of stakeholder participation and involving patient groups directly in each of its drug appraisals. With yet more citizen participation being signalled in the NHS Plan, the final item in the section discussing this read:

> A new Citizens Council will be established to advise the National Institute for Clinical Excellence on its clinical assessments. It will complement the work of the NICE Partners Council which provides a forum for the health service and industry to comment on the work of NICE. (DH, 2000: para 10.34)

The Citizens Council sat four-square in the move towards new, inclusive, participatory government practices described above. Commentators at the time saw it as pivotal for the further development of citizen participation. It was "a potentially radical model for public involvement" (Clarke, 2002: 35). It was alone, suggested the authors of a five-country review of healthcare rationing and priority setting, in pioneering national level citizen involvement, and as such could well come to serve as an exemplar of a necessary new synthesis between expert and lay inputs (Ham and Robert, 2003: 10-11, 151). But just how would it work? Would it embody the contradictions and suffer the fate of some of the other national level initiatives described earlier in this chapter? In many ways, it was still a step into the unknown. It had to be a matter of wait and see (Coulter, 2002: 5).

Conclusion

Writing in 2002, Robin Clarke was convinced that "more effort is being put into involving the public in decision making than at any previous time" (Clarke, 2002: 40). We have witnessed a continuing rise of citizen participation since that time. Participation is a theme that thoroughly infuses contemporary political debates in the UK. It has spread across sectors and across jurisdictions. The potential for involving the public in building a consensus around rationing services in health, for example, has been debated in continental Europe, in the US and in Australia and New Zealand (Ham and Robert, 2003). Citizen participation in health policy has had a high profile in the Netherlands and in the Scandinavian countries (Tritter: forthcoming). Debates about finding effective ways to engage citizens in political decision making will almost certainly outlive the specific party programmes with which they are associated at any one time.

Drawing on recent policy developments in the UK, this chapter has highlighted some of the contradictions that emerge from this growing desire to create direct citizen participation. Three points can be singled out. First, enthusiasm for participation has tended to obscure more careful thinking about what can be achieved. Policy frameworks remain ambiguous about the 'why?', the 'who?' and the 'how?' of citizen participation. Mixed expectations ensue, and the potential for disillusion is high. Second, efforts to involve citizens at local level have run ahead of those to involve them nationally. More than one national level initiative of late has run into the ground. Several reasons for this have been suggested. Asking people to take part at a local level where the matter is of immediate consequence to them as residents, for example, may be easier than asking them to discuss an abstract-seeming issue calling on a more nebulous identity as citizen. Third, questions of power and control stalk this field. Under what conditions can citizen participation become truly empowering for citizens? And how can its results be reconciled with practices of accountability of local and national governments and their agents? All of these issues are ones that will recur through the pages of this book.

Finally, there is a vitally important distinction to be made between stakeholder participation and citizen participation. A stakeholder dialogue starts with the premise that there are legitimate, pre-established positions and interests, and that these need to come to the table in an open way to be confronted, negotiated and reconciled. A dialogue between citizens, by contrast, starts with a premise of shared identity as members of a polity. The quest as citizens is to find a course of action contributing to the common good. How are they to ensure that relevant differences are revealed and accommodated appropriately within their discussions? The answer that is increasingly put forward is that citizens must 'deliberate'. Just what deliberation means in this context, and what kind of demands it makes on those designing and populating an assembly of citizens, is the subject for the next chapter.

TWO

Deliberation: towards an understanding of practice

Consider a sentence that opens as follows: 'As a result of the committee's deliberations, we have concluded...'. Such a sentence is more likely to be written than spoken. The phrase is less likely to come from the lips of a politician than from those of a public figure, respected and deemed independent. It is still likely — although perhaps a little less so than in the past — that the speaker will be white and will be male. Invoking the word deliberation in this context conjures not only a 'who?' but also a 'how?' question. We are invited to picture the committee's exchanges as cool and calm, as exchanges that will have involved careful and respectful listening and the weighing and balancing of competing arguments. The implied contrast is with what we might call 'normal' political debate. Here participants are clearly positioned in the argument and have an eye to the interests that they represent. They are often seemingly angry and emotional, and they are frequently keen to demolish not only the arguments but also the person of their 'opponents'.

Theorists of democratic deliberation and deliberative democracy both draw on, and distance themselves from, political debate construed in this way. They envisage a politics where there is well-informed reflection and argumentation on the part of a much wider citizenry, who are both prepared and able to engage. This chapter will examine debates about deliberation and explore some of the practical questions that arise when efforts are made to put deliberation into practice. The concern is not so much with the notion of a deliberative democracy and how its various institutions might dovetail with each other, but rather with the possibility of a *practice* of democratic deliberation. Chapter One charted the rising interest in and demand for citizen participation in policy making, highlighting some of the practical and political difficulties that Labour governments faced after 1997, when they tried to instigate such practices. How far does current theory illuminate the problems they faced? How does it need to be developed in order to carry out the in-depth empirical studies that, as we shall see, the theoretical analysts now feel are necessary if understanding is to go further?

The chapter is in four parts. The first part offers a brief introduction to some key theoretical debates. While these are often centred on an ideal form of deliberation, we can also trace a growing interest in practical matters of how to design deliberation and embed it in actual practice – something, not surprisingly, which has begun to modify the deliberative ideal. The next section focuses largely on experiments with citizens' juries. There are two reasons for this. In the first place, as Chapter One has indicated, such juries are very much to the fore in the policy community in the UK. In the second place, these represent the single most studied form of 'real world' deliberative assembly. Both the techniques for studying them and the lessons that are learned from them are thus relevant. The third section returns to the theoretical debates, identifying four major sets of objections to the deliberative ideal, and highlighting some of the considerations that a more adequate theory of deliberation needs to address. All this suggests that there is now a pressing need for a much more detailed ethnographic investigation than has been available hitherto. The final section develops a methodology and conceptual framework for such a study. It focuses on deliberation as a discursive activity and as an emergent form of social practice. It situates this approach in contemporary strands of theorising in sociology and social psychology, emphasising its value in addressing issues raised in the chapter, and setting out a series of specific research questions. The scene is thus set for the case study examined in Part II. The chapter starts, however, with the question, understood in terms of the debates which have dominated thinking in this area thus far: just what is deliberation and how has it been understood?

Deliberative ideal

As Chapter One has demonstrated, debates about democratic renewal that incorporate ideas about citizen deliberation (in a more or less precise way) are very much part of the contemporary political scene. Such debates, however, have also animated the discipline of political science in its explorations of changing relations between the state and civil society. Theoreticians have sought to address what they see as the simultaneous triumph and vulnerability of democracy in modern times (Hirst and Khilnani, 1996), and there has been a long-standing tradition exploring the potential for a more participatory politics (Pateman, 1976), developed, for example, through 'strong democracy' (Barber, 1984), 'associative democracy' (Hirst, 1994) and related ideas. For those grappling with issues such as these, the concept of a deliberative foundation for democracy has two potential attractions. In the first place, there is the aggregation of preferences issue. Voting relies on making a selection from a given set of options, and democratic choice comes down to a majority count derived from the simple aggregation of preferences. The voting process gives no indication either of the reasoning that underpins individual decisions or of the strength of feeling involved. Processes, furthermore, that might transform preferences rather than simply aggregate them are not available (Elster, 1998; Saward, 2000). This raises the question of whether democracy could not be more direct and more participatory. Second, there is the adversarial problem noted in the introduction to this chapter. Could democratic debate not manage to explore the nuances of a complex issue more, and to be less of a battle between pre-established preferences and positions? Reflecting on such dissatisfactions, Saward (2000: 5) puts matters concisely. Democracy must be more than 'just counting heads':

> It must involve discussions on an equal and inclusive basis, which deepen participants' knowledge of issues, awareness of the interests of others and the confidence to play an active part in public affairs.

There are some who find reasons to reject the deliberative turn out of hand (Sanders, 1997; Price, 2000). For most, however, the notion has a strong normative appeal. It seems to be inclusive and anti-elitist. It celebrates citizen potential and citizen capacity. It is profoundly optimistic in holding out hope for social solidarity, legitimacy and better decision making. However, we need to examine the idea of deliberation a little more closely.

To begin, it is helpful to take a step back. Theorists of deliberation frequently find their roots in two related traditions. First, there is the work of political philosopher John Rawls in his concern with justice, and in his attempt to identify 'public reason' and the 'precepts of reasonable discussion' (1971, 1997). By inviting us to imagine interacting under a 'veil of ignorance' as to how decisions will affect us, we can begin to see how ground rules for such a discussion might be devised and how an agreement might be reached by a group of participants whose individual interests in an outcome are diverse. Second, there is the work of sociologist and philosopher Jürgen

Habermas (1984, 1987, 1996). Drawing a contrast between (overextended) instrumental rationality oriented to the achievement of a given end, and (underdeveloped) communicative rationality oriented to understanding and mutual agreement, he outlines characteristics of a theory of communicative action. In what he terms an ideal speech situation, free and equal individuals come together in the public sphere in pursuit of a 'communicatively rational' agreement, one that persuades diverse participants and is capable of legitimating the exercise of political authority.

Drawing on these traditions, characterisations of democratic deliberation converge around a number of points. Deliberation entails a dialogue between people from different backgrounds who exchange thoughts about the issue, offer up reasons why others might be persuaded by a course of action, and reflect on the differences which emerge in the group. Participants consider jointly what – in the circumstances now revealed – might be said to be the most just course of action, or the one leading to the greatest public good. Their discussions are accompanied by the provision of a balanced range of information about relevant facts and values. The topic itself is usually of public interest and one where there is already lively controversy. The outcome of a process of public deliberation conceived in this way can be formulated in hypothetical terms. It is: *what a diverse group would come to think, if it were exposed to fact and opinion and given an opportunity to explore both of these in the light of the different interests that might be affected.*

Several advantages have been proposed for deliberation conceived in this way. One is that it produces better decisions through widening the range of considerations on the table and enhancing the likelihood of novel solutions. Others are: that it produces a superior result compared with polling (less a 'gut reaction' and more what people would think after informed reflection); and that it adds legitimacy to an eventual decision (Edelenbos and Klijn, 2004; cf Stirling, 2005). Claims have also been advanced for positive impacts on the citizens involved (motivating them towards public service, enhancing understanding of hard choices, and instilling community mindedness), as well as for potentially negative impacts. All the points here are ones that will recur, both in this chapter and later in the book.

For the present, however, it is worth dwelling on some of the presuppositions contained in such a notion of deliberation. Analytically at least there are three different moments in a deliberation. There is the exchange of initial views based on reasoning about one's position and experience as far as that can be articulated. There is a process of jointly digesting and reflecting on information made available (which may lead to changes of mind). And there are other-regarding exchanges – where participants consider the public good and offer reasons why others might change their minds. There is a strong requirement in all three moments that participants, while exploring the possibility of consensus, remain respectful of difference. There is the possibility that, if worldviews are incompatible and "reasonable people can disagree" (Cohen, 1998: 187), a group may find itself unable to arrive at a shared position. The outcome of deliberation in this instance is not a recommendation for a course of action but an account of the reasoning underpinning the different conclusions of those present.

Implicit within the description above is the much-cited requirement, stemming from concepts of the Habermasian ideal speech situation, that dialogue be "free from domination, coercion, manipulation and strategizing" so that "the only power remaining is that of better argument" (see, for example, Dryzek, 2000: 81; see also Budge, 2000: 200). The practical impossibility of this is widely acknowledged, but so too is the point that its statement as an ideal can help to identify what it is important to try to build in to the design of institutions and practices that seek to produce deliberation (Cohen, 1998).

Political scientists have worked with these ideas in diverse ways and with different emphases. They have also, however, been notable in making a move, or attracting others to make a move, towards practical institutional design. Two issues can be briefly discussed and serve to give a first flavour of 'real life' experiments with deliberation. First there is the question of information. Ideal deliberation, as described above, requires that relevant information (facts, values and opinions) is available, and is taken into account by participants in the deliberative process. How is this to be accomplished? The planning cells model (see Box 2.1), takes a largely *educative* approach, stressing the extent of learning and digesting of technical information and value positions that needs to take place. This can be contrasted with a citizens' jury model, where, as the metaphor would suggest, a somewhat more *interrogatory* approach is taken, relying on 'witnesses' who speak more explicitly in defence of different positions. (A later section of the chapter gives more detail on juries.) Clearly there is potential for contention around the nature and balance of information to be presented. Box 2.2 outlines another educative model example, where very considerable resources of both time and money were allocated to the business of collating and ordering information before deliberation began.

Box 2.1: The 'planning cells' model

Originating in Germany in 1972, and sponsored initially by the University of Wuppertal, planning cells comprise randomly selected groups of citizens working in parallel to tackle a predefined problem, over a time-limited period. Around 25 people, drawn from a specific geographical area, meet for between three and five days. They start by receiving written information, attending lectures and perhaps making site visits. This 'curriculum' is divided into basic and agreed facts, interpretations of facts (where all significant viewpoints are represented), and expert beliefs. Participants attend both 'lectures' and 'hearings' where witnesses cover the range of views. They then discuss options and likely consequences. Much work is performed in small groups of about five people. A neutral facilitator is provided and an alternative can be requested. Values are tapped through questionnaires and group discussions. In some cases multi-attribute utility theory is used to create a matrix of relative weights and utility values on each criterion. The facilitator prepares the report, which is fed back to participants before being released. A feature of the model is that there are multiple groups, up to two dozen, meeting in different locations on the same topic. Urban planning has been a major focus for planning cells in Germany, the first of which related to a waste disposal facility. In 20 years, 26 towns adopted this method. In the period up to 1995 there were at least four examples of planning cells on national topics, one, for example, on alternative energy policies.

Source: Dienel and Renn (1995)

Box 2.2: The 'great debate' model

Following a deadlock on siting nuclear power plants, the Dutch Parliament agreed to a wide-ranging national debate on energy policy. The question to be debated was to be broad-based, there was to be participation in selecting the model of participation, an accessible information base and attention to norms, values and interests – with a focus on value reconciliation. A steering committee consulted widely on the rules and agenda. There was a staff of 30 and a total budget of $15 million (1980 prices). An information phase covered production of an inventory of opinions and arguments. There were regional hearings, open invitations to comment and 'controversy sessions' (open to the public) to explore whether divergences of opinion could be reduced.

Specific studies were commissioned to plug information gaps. Funds were allocated to train moderators and to subsidise less well-resourced groups to enable them to take part. An interim report served as a common database for the main discussion phase. This included a questionnaire used in over 1,800 local discussion groups, with locally hired discussion leaders, another 1,100 discussions in schools, trades unions etc, and a further 300-plus political organisations, commercial companies and interest groups who were also asked for an opinion. A 400-page final report was prepared covering the whole process. There were earlier examples of similar initiatives in Sweden, France and Austria.

Sources: Midden (1995); Mumpower (1995)

If information is one major practical challenge, representation is another. On what basis should citizens make their appearance in a deliberative arena? And can they be said to be representative of citizens in general? In principle, all should have an equal chance of recruitment, and in local settings random selection using the electoral roll, or stratified random sampling to ensure that diverse groups are represented in what is a small gathering of sometimes only 10 or 12 deliberators, is often used. Repeat deliberations, as in both models described above, serve to widen coverage and lend greater statistical acceptability of results. Deliberative opinion polling, a technique particularly associated with the name of political scientist James Fishkin, is another method that can draw in large numbers. Beginning with a survey of a random population sample, members attend a weekend of briefing and discussions after which they are polled again to establish changes of view. Numbers involved have ranged from 200 to more than 450. Originating in the US, deliberative polling has been used in Australia, Denmark and the UK (Fishkin, 1995; Fishkin and Luskin, 2000). Deliberative techniques nonetheless remain vulnerable to the charge of lack of representativeness; many would acknowledge that another group on another day might well come to produce different results. This often leads commissioning organisations to conclude that they should treat recommendations not as conclusive but as one kind of evidence to be set alongside others – thus leaving existing mechanisms of accountability intact.

Far and away the most popular model of deliberation, however, is that of the citizens' jury. The concept of the jury, examples of its implementation, and the body of commentary and research assessment that it has attracted, provide themes for the next section.

Deliberation in action – 'jury style'

The concept of citizens' juries was first devised more than 40 years ago in Europe and the US in the context of concerns about democratic renewal. More than a dozen juries had been conducted in the US by the early 1990s (see Box 2.3), when the idea was picked up by the IPPR, a UK think-tank, again with the intention of further strengthening democracy (Stewart et al, 1994). Over a two-year period, IPPR conducted five pilot juries, all in the field of health (Coote and Lenaghan, 1997). Subsequently, three more pilot juries in health were initiated by the King's Fund (McIver, 1998). There were others under the auspices of the Local Government Management Board (LGMB, 1996). By 2001, at least 100 citizens' juries had taken place in the UK (Wakeford, 2002) on subjects ranging from Northern Ireland, to education reform, waste disposal, healthcare and genetic testing (for some examples, see Dunkerley and Glasner, 1998; Barnes, 1999; Petts, 2001).

Box 2.3 gives a description of the key elements of procedure in the original model. This has not always been followed to the letter. In the US, practicalities often meant that the oversight committee element was dropped and, in the UK in particular, local councils and health authorities often used the jury in a rapid, one-off form rather than allowing for repeat juries on the original parallel juries/two-stage model. 'Do-It-Yourself' (DIY) juries offer a variant designed as a response to the perceived danger of sponsor capture (Wakeford, 2002). Here jury members set the question themselves, summon witnesses of their own choosing and it is they alone who put the final report and recommendations together. DIY juries also employ an oversight panel where stakeholders ensure that a balance of information and expertise is available and that the recommendations are taken forward into the policy arena.

Both initiators and those given the task of evaluation suggest that juries have both significance and strong advantages (Stewart et al, 1994; Crosby, 1995; Davies et al, 1998). Introducing an account that distils a wealth of detail about IPPR's five juries on health topics, for example, Coote and Lenaghan (1997) see these as a potential way forward for a more 'mature' relationship between state and citizen. In an overview, they conclude that juries can certainly handle complex issues, and they argue that "there is far more enthusiasm, ability and 'community spirit' among ordinary citizens than most decision-makers routinely assume" (p 90). While they acknowledge that the time and cost commitments are high, that more refinements

Box 2. 3: Citizens' juries

Citizens' juries were first developed by an independent agency, the Jefferson Center for New Democratic Processes, in the US in 1974. According to the original model, citizens' juries are selected with the aim of providing a microcosm of the population at large to discuss and give their view on a particular policy issue. A jury consists of 12-24 members, who are paid to attend hearings over 4-5 days, and at which witnesses – selected by an independent group or by jurors themselves – present different points of view. A very direct, short and clear topic or 'charge' is given by a sponsoring agency and worked up by staff. A neutral moderator is available to facilitate all sessions, but jurors have an opportunity to work in private, and a chance to review and finally approve any recommendations that emerge. Ideally an Oversight Committee of former jurors reviews the rules and staff performance and is important in ensuring that staff do not dominate, but funding has not always been available for it. In the US such citizens' juries were held locally and nationally. Early juries were regionally based and considered environmental and health topics and issues for elections. The first ones were two-stage – five parallel juries sending representatives forward to a further one.

Sources: Armour (1995); Crosby (1995)

to the method are indicated and that much still depends on the skill of the moderators, their overall conclusions remain very positive. McIver (1998), assessing the NHS juries sponsored by the King's Fund, is another largely positive evaluator. Her interviews suggested that all of those involved felt that participants understood issues sufficiently to make practical and useful recommendations. As in the previous case, she observes that the jurors themselves found the experience rewarding. She concludes that citizens' juries can be an effective vehicle in enabling local people to have a positive impact on policy decisions. A more recent contribution has gone further, and suggested that juries can sometimes find ways out of a political deadlock (Parkinson, 2004a). Pickard (1998), examining two juries convened and hosted by a single health authority, is less sanguine, however. She warns that different styles of facilitation and different ways of questioning witnesses can shape recommendations. She spends considerable time on the question of independence and control, arguing ultimately that citizens' juries should not be "elevated beyond the rank of other methods of public involvement"

(Pickard, 1998: 242) and she opts in the end for deliberative polling as a preferable technique.

In practice, some of the strongest criticisms focus on questions of jury independence and, in particular, on links with formal, political accountability for decisions. We have already seen the divergence of views in the UK between those in local government who see citizens' juries as advisory only, and some in the science community calling for public consultation to be directly consequential. Cheyne and Comrie (2002) recount an example in New Zealand, where Wellington City Council convened a citizens' jury to consider the future of their electricity supplier. Despite acceptance that the jury process was well and fairly conducted, the mayor rejected the jury's conclusion and the Council was not prepared to revisit its conclusions in the light of the citizens' jury's opinion. Hendriks (2002), in an Australian example, highlights the additional unease that can be generated among established interest groups, when a new public participation forum is added to the political mix. Williams (2004) cautions that officials, in his case local government officials, need to make very clear the limits to the powers that they have to effect change, and how much they may or may not be able to take on the conclusions of a citizens' jury. Wakeford (2002), in an updating newsletter, offers a wry comment that "some suspect that citizens' juries have sometimes been used as show-trials that allow those in power to avoid engaging in processes that might hold them accountable to communities".

This raises the question of the independence of citizens' juries and the extent to which – wittingly or not – they are open to influence and manipulation by those who design and run the events. Smith, working in the field of environmental issues and green politics, provides a series of discussions of this (Smith and Wales, 2000; Smith, 2001, 2003), emphasising just how important factors such as the nature of the facilitation and the selection of witnesses and information can be. He also draws on Dryzek's (2000) concern about a lack of opportunity for oppositional discourses to emerge in state-sponsored deliberative forums. And, in what is an important parallel stream of work in science studies (see Chapter One), Stirling offers a particularly salutary summary on the multiple ways in which the design and implementation of a deliberative process can have unintended effects:

> Relationships with sponsors, the constitution of oversight, the design of the process, the choice of focus, the

partitioning of perspectives, the engagement of stakeholders, the recruitment of participants, the phrasing of questions, the bounding of remits, the characterizing of alternatives, the provision of information, the medium of discourse, the conduct of facilitation, the demeanour of practitioners, the personalities of protagonists, the dynamics of deliberation, the management of dissension, the documentation of findings, the articulation of policy – all provide ample scope for contingent variability, inadvertent bias or the exercise of deliberate conditioning influence. (Stirling, 2005: 225)

One strand of recent work has begun to focus on alternative institutional designs for citizen participation, their merits and demerits. Work carried out for an independent inquiry into the state of democracy in Britain, commissioned to explore new democratic forms, identified as many as a dozen different designs for deliberation. It concluded that these have advantages when compared with more traditional ways of consulting the public, but noted too that they have considerable resource implications and that independent facilitation is vital. Both compared with each other and with other kinds of democratic innovations (referendums, for example, co-governance, direct democracy and e-democracy), all had advantages and disadvantages. No single method stood out as preferable in all circumstances (Smith, 2005). Thompson and Hoggett (2001) bring group analytic theory to bear, with its focus on the emotional dynamics inherent in a deliberative arena, to argue that while ignoring these can subvert or destroy deliberative spaces, sensitivity to them can allow them to be harnessed in support of better deliberation. Stokkom (2005), while challenging the theoretical underpinning, takes forward the new classificatory work, distinguishing between stakeholder committees and citizens' fora (cf Smith, 2001), and going on to identify a series of possible power and emotional dynamics in each. Also of interest in the present context is the work of Barnes and her colleagues. This focuses on limitations in how 'the public' is constituted for deliberation – both in the design and the process of participatory practices (Barnes et al, 2003) – and crucially emphasises the need for styles of activity that bring difference into deliberation (Barnes, 2002). All this begins to bring empirical work into more direct engagement with the critics of deliberation, whose arguments are discussed in the following section.

What, in sum, has empirical work on deliberation in action added?

The literature has shifted from advocacy to more independent evaluative commentary. It has also begun to move from domination by pragmatic, 'what works?' evaluations to rather more theoretically driven work. The ideal of deliberative reasoning is operationalised in a fairly loose way and the focus, it seems, is beginning to polarise. Some of the work noted above has begun to suggest that literatures in social psychology might offer a way forward in deepening understanding of the dynamics of the deliberative event. Other work urges that we attend much more to contingencies in the design of a deliberative initiative, and look to traditions in organisational analysis for further enlightenment. Can these be brought together in some way? Is a more adequate socio-psychological theory of deliberation now possible – one that would respond to the call for an 'expanded' notion of dialogue (Barnes, 2004: 131) that some of the critics are now demanding? Before turning to these questions, it is important to take a closer look at what some of the theorists have said, not about the ideal of deliberation but about the process of deliberating.

Dilemmas in deliberating

Debates in political science around deliberation are now legion. Critics in the main are sympathetic to the ideal, but raise problems with the attempt to render it operational. This section selects four related challenges from this corpus of work, providing a critical re-examination with an eye towards what they might mean for developing a theoretically informed, in-depth examination of deliberation in practice.

Power, pluralism and oppression

Deliberators, so the conventional argument goes, need to act as equals. If they are to engage with each other effectively, power differences need to be neutralised in the interests of full debate. One view is that active facilitation (including reminders about the common good, direct encouragement of quieter participants and routine invitations to offer a different view) pushes in this direction. Another is that the very process of reasoning in public will help to temper dominant voices and encourage the more reticent to speak out. A debate on pluralism takes this further by asking whether there are some positions that participants will bring that must be ruled out because they eclipse and oppress others – whether, in other words, deliberation can work as pure 'process' or whether it must be accompanied by substantive rules about justice (see Gutman and Thompson, 2002). The case of the 'white man from Arizona', drawn from practical experience of deliberative polling, provides a process-oriented take on this. In a deliberation on family issues he challenged the black, female, single parent woman from New York, arguing that her situation could not be counted as a 'family' at all. Much later in the process, he approached her to say "I was wrong" (Fishkin and Luskin, 2000: 26). Inspiring as the illustration is, we do not know what induced the man from Arizona to change his mind. Nor, and equally importantly, do we know what prompted the woman from New York to stay and presumably to continue to offer interventions from a standpoint that he had refused to acknowledge.

The underlying problem here is that of hegemonic discourse and its power to legitimate inequalities. Iris Young (2000: 108) offers a warning:

> Under circumstances of structural social and economic inequality, the relative power of some groups often allows them to dominate the definition of the common good in ways compatible with their experience, perspective and priorities. A common consequence of social privilege is the ability of a group to convert its perspective in some issues into authoritative knowledge without being challenged by those who have reason to see things differently.

The simple granting of presence to a subordinated group is not enough (Phillips, 1995). Young (1989) is known for a proposal that members of such a group need to meet in sameness before they can articulate difference. Concerns about the potential of deliberation to undermine a citizen's sense of self and promote an identity at odds with experience (Stokes, 1998) have their roots here. Any adequate theorising of deliberation must address the resources that citizens bring to a deliberative arena, the way in which these are already colonised by hegemonic discourses and the circumstances under which oppositional positions may be successfully articulated. Such an approach, as we begin to suggest later, is likely to involve further development of theories of power.

Arguing from interests

Interests occupy a complex place in political science thinking about deliberation. On the one hand, deliberation aims ultimately to set interests aside and to reason about the common good:

> ... citizens treat one another as equals not by giving equal consideration to interests ... but by offering them justifications for the exercise of collective power framed in terms of considerations that can, roughly speaking, be acknowledged by all as reasons. (Cohen, 1998: 186)

On the other hand, interests cannot be so easily set aside in the context of a deliberative process. Once again Young is helpful. Communication from different perspectives, she argues, acts as a corrective to partial views and "enables a public collectively to construct a more comprehensive account of how social processes work and therefore of the likely consequences of proposed policies" (Young, 2000: 83). Good deliberators thus need to acknowledge that they are together in a single political space; they need to be committed to naming and trying to work out potential conflicts of interest in a peaceable way (Young, 2000: 110).

There is a further complication. Formal and organised interests (of capital and labour, of environmental lobbyists and so on) that have a place in pluralist politics are often quite specifically ruled out of a deliberative arena. Mainstream political science theorising envisages citizens coming to a deliberative event as citizens rather than lobbyists. Practical initiatives often reflect this, choosing deliberators in ways that reflect demographic diversity and sometimes placing those with an interest in a separate, stakeholder discussion arena. What this fails to acknowledge is the problematic place that is thereby constructed for the personal experience of deliberators. Barnes (2004) addresses this. Drawing from her own and others' empirical research involving older people, for example, and mental health survivors, her argument is that room must be made both for affect and for what professionals and policy makers often dismiss as 'anecdote'. This, in effect, blurs the boundary between deliberation as a model of citizen participation as conceived here, and forms of participation of service users. Without necessarily taking this road, it remains vitally important to acknowledge that the interests that deliberators have will be opaque. They will arise in complex ways as a result of life experience and the intersection of this with social positioning in terms of age, gender, class, ethnicity and other factors. Effective theorising about deliberation must thus address the multiple identities that are mobilised in a deliberative arena and the ways in which speaking from a position as a mother, a worker, a resident, a person with a disability and so on, is accomplished (see Squires, 1998; Barnes et al, 2003: 383).

Knowledge, expertise and experience

Deliberation needs to be informed by relevant kinds of knowledge. Central to current theorising is the claim that citizens must make a transition from an entirely understandable position of "rational ignorance" on many topics (Fishkin and Luskin, 2000: 18) to becoming the "engaged and informed public" that deliberation requires. There is hence an issue both of making alternative knowledge available, and of using varied discursive styles; drama, anecdote, role-play and the individual case can at times help participants to understand what is at stake. Commentators frequently recognise the danger of capture. 'Informed' decision making too easily collapses into 'manipulated' decision making (Smith and Wales, 1999: 305) if the selection of informants is skewed; models that bring a diverse stakeholder group into the process to confirm that information is balanced can go some way towards mitigating this. Bang and Dryberg (2000: 147), however, put a further issue firmly on the table here, in terms of giving warrant to direct challenges to mainstream scientific expertise. They object that in current practice the possibility of connecting lay experience and scientific expertise is "ruled out from the outset". They insist:

> What we need is a model of deliberation that allows for self-governance and identity-formation on the part of both experts and lay actors, and which moreover recognizes that co-governance between them requires acceptance of their differences with regard to their individuality and commonality.

This is an argument that has been picked up in particular in the world of science studies. One issue, already noted in Chapter One, is to do with making space at an early stage for questions that are outside the frame of experts. Another is the need to develop the 'interactional expertise' that allows citizens to interrogate those differently positioned in an expert debate (Collins and Evans, 2002). Despite its rooting in critical theory drawing on Habermas' concern to devise ways to challenge narrow notions of scientific rationality, the problem of deference towards expertise and the danger that oppositional discourses may be crowded out (Dryzek, 2000a) remains. Further empirical work must be demonstrably alert to the conditions under which critical engagement with expertise can occur.

'Sanitised' debates or messy practice?

Just how feasible is it to expect that interaction between citizens could generate deliberation in the sense defined earlier of informed and other-regarding debate across difference? Is the deliberative ideal 'unrealistically sanitised'? Is it modelling itself on the university seminar – making a move that tries, in effect, to "take the politics out of politics" (Budge, 2000: 200)? In related vein, Johnson (1998: 166) asks: "should we banish not only obstreperous demands and angry shouts, but tears and laughter from the deliberative arena?". Dryzek is one theorist who has had a change of heart on this. "The only condition for authentic deliberation," he suggests, is "that communication [should] induce reflection upon preferences in non-coercive fashion" (Dryzek, 2000a: 1-2).

Young goes further. In conditions of inequality, inclusion requires that different modes of discourse be utilised in redeeming contributions to the debate. Her work on public 'greeting' (that is, acknowledging others), on rhetoric and on narrative as key conditions of inclusive dialogue addresses this, and she warns that unless we recognise varied forms of argument, the possibilities for deliberation may be unduly restricted (Young, 2000: 56). The strong position taken by Barnes on the inclusion of affect and anecdote has already been noted. Task-based and problem-solving forums, she warns, "can close down the opportunities for developing understanding and valuing diverse experiences and styles" (Barnes, 2004: 131). She suggests that it is the discomfort of professionals and policy makers with expressions of passion and pain that disallows other possibilities. Points such as these are a reminder that the picture on the ground will be complex. Deliberation as such will only take up some proportion of a deliberative event. And what counts as deliberative activity has extended. Any new conceptual scheme needs to encompass not just the other-regarding 'reasonable' exchanges in the basic model, but the recognition and challenge of 'unreasonable' sentiments where these occur. It also needs to pay attention to just how discursive devices such as humour, gossip and stories function to demolish positions as well as to explore and reconcile them.

What conclusions can be drawn? To date, the obvious route for theoretically informed empirical enquiry about deliberation has been to measure against an 'ideal mode of argument' yardstick derived from Habermas or Rawls. Webler (1995) provides the most direct example, utilising a set of criteria developed from his own reading of Habermas on communicative rationality, and urging collaborators to present case study material in direct relation to his schema (Renn et al, 1995). No strong body of work has emerged subsequently which takes such a route, and the discussion in this chapter has started to move in a rather different direction. It has identified difficulties of contesting hegemonic discourse and of engaging critically with expertise; it has stressed the importance of understanding the mobilisation and legitimation of multiple identities, and the point that actual deliberation is always likely to be messier than the model. Considerations such as these provide the starting point for the new framework for empirical research outlined below. It is then exemplified in action in Part II of the book and further developed in Part III. Drawing in particular from developments in discourse studies, the approach makes a decisive shift away from appeals to a pre-given abstract model of deliberation towards a more 'bottom-up' orientation to forms of social practice.

Developing a framework for research

As explained in the Introduction to this book, an opportunity to address deliberation in close-up came for the present authors in the autumn of 2002, when we were commissioned to evaluate the Citizens Council being set up by the National Institute of Clinical Excellence (NICE). The intention of the Institute was to create an assembly in which 'ordinary citizens' could debate issues with which NICE was involved. The aim was to tease out what members of the public would think, were they to be exposed to relevant information, and given a chance to explore and discuss together. The research was to address 'how best to make use of citizens' time, when members of the public are invited to discuss complex issues'. More specifically, it was to examine the process of recruitment and selection, the rationale for the choice of topics and the processes determining these. We were enjoined to assess whether the Citizens Council members felt they were well supported and how they perceived their role. We were to investigate how Council reports were produced and received within the Institute. Most particularly, however, we were to examine the actual conduct of the meetings as these developed over a two-year period. An *ethnographic* study was wanted.

This provided an opportunity for a much closer observation of deliberation in action than had been yet available in the literature. Using video-recordings and transcribing the dialogue of the Council would give us an unprecedented database on deliberation in action. We would be able to explore the nature of the discursive resources that participants brought to bear, to examine the different forms and styles of interaction, teasing out and assessing the ways in which information was handled and power relations were enacted. By following a succession of meetings, we could make a start on identifying features of the event design that facilitated deliberation and those which constrained it. We could also go beyond a micro-analysis. The terms of the research commission were such that we were invited into the sponsoring organisation; we would have access to the rationales that shaped the design of the Council, and to the people and events that would influence the reception of the work of the Council. In short, the chance was there to explore deliberation and address some of the fundamental issues raised by democratic deliberation and citizen participation in a new way.

Case studies (even those with a longitudinal element) have disadvantages. The degree to which the findings can be generalised to other contexts is limited. But they have one major advantage when a field of research is 'top-heavy' with theory and 'in principle' abstract specifications, as arguably is the case for academic discussions of deliberation. A detailed case study provides a concrete actuality. If we could show, in a fine-grain way, some of the patterns in practice, a clearer sense might emerge of how to conceptualise deliberation as a set of participant activities. If we could understand the translation process as policy is devised and then enacted through an organisation we might have a clearer view of the organisational and policy challenges and go beyond formulations of sponsor capture. In the first instance, what was required was an evaluation study with a strong formative element. This completed (Davies et al, 2005), there was material in abundance to go on to address the kinds of questions set out in this chapter and to engage with the question of a new stage of theory development in relation to citizen deliberation.

Social practices and communities of practice

Guiding the development of the present ethnography have been the twin concepts of deliberation as social practice and the Citizens Council as a community of practice. Social practice approaches are helpful in making sense of the highly open, fluid and contingent nature of deliberation, as revealed in the empirical studies of citizens' juries and other initiatives, and are capable of addressing the multiple levels of complex interaction likely to be involved. Theorists of practice (Bourdieu, 1977, 1990; Giddens, 1979; Schatzki et al, 2001; Warde, 2004) allow for multiple contingencies, but they also accept that regularities start to become apparent.

Authors in this tradition define social practices as coordinated activities and performances which bring new situations into being but which are constrained by, in interaction with, and sometimes in tension with, surrounding practices and with what has gone before. While practice in general is not strictly determined or governed by rules, the unfolding of any particular practice shows regularities and routines, and depends on, and reproduces, familiar procedures continually customised and worked up for new contexts. Such activity involves both social, often institutionalised, actions together with territory demarcated as psychological – the minds, emotions, motivations, cognitions and personalities of social actors. Practice is collective (dependent on the articulation of shared resources). It is also about reflexive transformation, setting new conditions for what is possible in the process of becoming (Giddens, 1979). Weick (2004), drawing on Taylor and van Every (2000), and working in the field of organisations, offers a metaphor of 'smoke and crystal'. Practice has some dispersed, swirling, fragile, dynamic and smoke-like features, but is not random. It can also be robust, highly predictable, solid and tight, without ever having the symmetry, 'endless' stability and 'thing-like' fixity of crystal. The 'logic of practice' in this sense lies between the crystal and the smoke.

A particularly notable advantage of the concept of social practice in the present context lies in its engagement with micro-, meso- and macro- levels of social organisation. It was clear that an understanding of the NICE Citizens Council would require work at all these levels. At the micro-level, there were the interactions that made up any particular moment in a Council meeting. Practice theory, however, stresses that these emerging micro-orders would be conditioned by higher order social practices (cf Cicourel, 1981). We could expect, therefore, that the emerging order coalescing around the design of the Council in the Institute would in turn be conditioned by the macro-policy contexts already sketched out in Chapter One. Box 2.4 draws out some simplified contrasts that serve to emphasise some of the philosophical commitments governing theories of practice, both demonstrating their roots in anti-foundationalism and social constructionism.

Box 2.4: The power of practice theorising

From order as regularities in norms and customs ... to order as arrangements of people, artefacts and things giving meaning to activity in fields of practice....

From order arising out of individual agency or constraining individual action ... to order as emerging in a field of practice, (re)constitutive of individuals, flexible and changeable....

From material contexts shaping order ... to materially interwoven practices and order as emerging from shared practical understandings....

From assumptions about individual mental states (beliefs, emotions...) to concepts of embodied capacities (know-how, skills, tacit understandings, dispositions)....

From the privileging of innate reason and rationality ... to the recognition of varying forms of reasoning and argumentation in different fields of practice....

From contrasts between macro- and micro-level analyses ... to intersecting practices, some anchoring and constraining others, some as existing in and through practice....

From theory as predictive and propositional ... to theory as more inductive, descriptive and open-ended....

The concept of communities of practice (Lave and Wenger, 1991; Wenger, 1999) puts further flesh on this thinking. A community of practice is a gathering of people whose activities are guided by their common purpose and whose joint goals and aims emerge through negotiated understandings among members. Unlike other concepts of community such as 'speech communities', 'discourse communities',

'communities of interest', 'communities of identity', 'rhetorical communities' and so on, a community of practice is defined in terms of the mutual engagement and situated learning that takes place among its members. Particularly important for our study is the notion of interlinked and sometimes clashing communities of practice. NICE, at the time of the research, was still fairly new, but it was an established organisation, and a key part of new governance arrangements devised by the political party in power. The Citizens Council was a group with 'zero history', although over time it was to acquire a history. In the analysis that follows in Part II, we present both the Institute and the Council as cohering sites of practice, where each is engaged in producing particular kinds of products using the communal resources members develop as they progress. These include: shared forms of knowledge, repertoires, artefacts, procedures, designs, documents, tools, narratives, apocryphal stories, telling anecdotes, ethical frames and so on. New communities of practice involve intensive and shared learning. As Eckert (2000) has elegantly demonstrated, over time, people in such a community develop and come to share ways of doing things – ways of talking and being together, modes of organising, identities and values as a consequence of their mutual engagement in their common task. The contributing semiotic worlds of individual members and subgroups begin to overlap and intertwine, producing new social practices. A key aim in what follows is to identify and describe these interwoven processes, including both the distinctive practices that came to constitute the Citizens Council, and those that guided NICE as the organisation sponsoring, shaping and hosting the initiative.

Discourse and practice

A study of social practices is also a study of discourse. Discourse became a core concept for an ethnography of deliberation not simply because human meaning making sets the horizon for any material or non-material activity (cf Laclau and Mouffe, 1987), but also because the practices under investigation are acts of communication and representation which work through talk and texts (Potter and Wetherell, 1987). All communities of practice make meaning. More than many communities of practice, however, deliberative initiatives are very directly about designing discursive environments. A deliberative forum is a space designed to encourage particular kinds of talk, and the products (reports and recommendations) further depend on complex discursive practices.

Discourse analysis (cf Wetherell et al, 2001a) offers an epistemological standpoint that chimes well with practice theorising. It entails a constructionist theory of meaning and an anti-foundationalist perspective on language. As Gergen (1985) has pointed out, the terms by which social actors account for the world are not dictated by the stipulated objects of such accounts. There can be no appeal to an objectivist understanding of a world independent of our collective formulations of it. The terms through which we achieve understanding are social artefacts, products of historically and culturally situated interchanges between people. This holds both for those we study and for our own accounts as analysts and theorists.

There are now, of course, many discourse theories and modes of discourse analysis for studying those constituting terms, and the organisation, negotiation and patterning of the interchanges and social artefacts emphasised by a constructionist standpoint (Wetherell et al, 2001b). The approach used for this study was strongly influenced by the ethnography of communication (Fitch, 2001), and drew on sociolinguistic discourse concepts such as speech situation and speech or discursive style (Cameron, 2001), as these allowed attention to broader patterns across what became a very large discourse corpus. The discursive analysis in Part II develops some simple pragmatic quantitative measures for tracking theoretically important discursive phenomena such as, for example, numbers of particular kinds of back-and-forth exchanges. Quantitative work allows a comparison across time, assessing the impact of issues of design. This is combined, however, with qualitative (but still relatively broad-brush) attention to discourse processes. We looked, for example, at positioning and genre, and tried to illustrate what deliberation looks like in practice as unfolding interaction. Although Part II gives a detailed account commensurate with our purposes, there is always more analysis that can be conducted. The corpus is such that future research on it can slice through it in different ways using other discourse methods and concepts.

It is a central aim of this book to demonstrate that discourse analysis has the capacity both to put flesh on the sometimes rather vague notion of practice, and to address the specific needs for development of deliberation theory identified earlier in the chapter. Discourse analysis provides a way of investigating in depth how 'the public' is constituted in the operation of a Citizens Council, as some work now directly recommends and has begun to explore

(Barnes et al, 2003: 396; see also Hodge, 2005). It can illuminate the various iconic and mythic figures and constructions which populate deliberation theory and which have become entangled with ideals on the ground. Also, a discursive perspective offers a generative theory of power, attending to the way power constructs issues and identities and in this way raising more thoroughgoing concerns about dominance and its operations than some of the more circumscribed anxieties around deception, strategising and influence highlighted by many critics of deliberation and described earlier in this chapter.

Discursive investigation also offers a way of linking the frames constructed within a sponsor organisation for a deliberative initiative, the organisational narratives that guide both the overall design of a deliberative event, and the micro-practices that serve to make up the day-to-day deliberations of the Council. Included here are the subject positions offered to citizens *in situ* as identities and taken up or resisted by them. Discourse analyses drawing on discursive psychology (Edwards and Potter, 1992) question notions of pre-existing interests and the reason–emotion splits and binaries that characterise very many discussions of deliberation. We can look also at the discursive reception of the fruits of deliberation both within and outside NICE. In short, the standpoint of discourse analysis, coupled with concepts from the field of social practice, has, we claim, the capacity to clarify afresh the field of democratic deliberation and to offer new insights on it.

Box 2.5 below sets out eight specific questions that have guided the case study presented in Part II of this book. Embedded in the answers to such questions are constructions of the citizen and host, notions of competence and capability, ideas about appropriate modes of conduct, expression and demeanour – all of which, as we shall see, become consequential for the practice and the outcome of deliberation.

Box 2.5: Research questions

1. What is the nature of the discursive environment in which a sponsor organisation makes sense of a deliberative initiative? What are the organisational narratives framing the context and constructing opportunities and constraints?

2. What forms of knowledge are mobilised by sponsors to design a deliberative assembly? How are ideas about recruitment and facilitation, for example, filtered through the organisation? What internal and external contingencies shape this?

3. What discursive practices develop in a deliberative assembly? What ways of engaging witnesses discussing issues and interacting emerge?

4. How is the nascent community of practice affected by design features? What facilitates and impedes deliberative engagement?

5. What does the process of becoming informed by experts do to citizen identity? What speaking positions and styles are available in relation to this?

6. How do issues of power, plural interests and hegemonic discourse raised by critics of the deliberative ideal play out in actual live contexts?

7. What are the elements that come to comprise a community of practice among deliberators? Which elements of prior structuring by the host organisation are accepted and which are resisted?

8. What are the spaces and mechanisms in which a host organisation seeks to manage the results of deliberation? How do these relate to differential understandings among its internal and external stakeholders? To what extent are they accepted or resisted by citizens in a deliberative assembly?

Conclusion

Deliberation, as it has been defined and explored in this chapter, involves discussion with a view to teasing out what a group would think, were it exposed to fact and opinion on a topic, and given a chance to explore and discuss together. Theoretical debates about deliberation make clear the complexity of this as a form of social interaction. It must inform without manipulating; it must give an equal voice to all who are present; and it must make space for new arguments, ones that counter hegemonic discourse, to be heard. More and more, the theoreticians have become interested in questions of institutional design, asking how deliberation can be made to work in practice. Politicians too, as we saw in Chapter One, are increasingly willing and anxious to find ways of enabling citizens' deliberation to occur.

In the light of this, we have argued for the need to develop a new kind of framework for empirical study. It must be one that does not seek in a mechanistic way to compare reality with an ideal, but is instead capable of handling complexity and contradiction, and of blending an understanding of both dynamics and design, and embedding deliberative initiatives more successfully in their contexts. Key elements in such a framework have now been outlined, based on contemporary theories of social practice, and utilising the conceptual tools of discourse analysis. With this in place, we are now in a position to turn, in Part II of this book, to the case study of NICE's Citizens Council.

Part II
A Citizens Council in action

THREE

Setting up a Citizens Council

> When people act they unrandomize variables, insert
> vestiges of orderliness, and literally create their own
> constraints. (Weick, 1979: 243)

New social practices are never entirely new. The 'vestiges of order'
that we insert into apparently novel situations and the constraints that
are thereby put in place serve to bring at least some familiar routines
into play. Furthermore, the process that Karl Weick (1995) was later to
call 'sense making' in organisations will be visible in the dialogues and
debates through which new practices start to crystallise and become
embedded. Exploring the unfolding of this in the meetings of the
Citizens Council of NICE is a major theme of the chapters that follow.
But sense making and creating constraints also had to be agreed and
accomplished in NICE as members of the Institute first set, and then
reset, parameters for the Council. To be sure, one constraint was already
given. As we saw in Chapter One, from the point of the political
announcement in the summer of 2001, there was to be a Citizens
Council. It was to work alongside the mechanisms of consultation
that the Institute already had in place. But the precise form it would
take and its ways of working remained to be settled.

The central concern of this chapter is with the first imagined shape
of the Council and the reasons why it took the form that it did. How
was the thinking within the Institute about a Citizens Council filtered
through its own understandings of itself and its ways of working?
How as a result of this was the Citizens Council given operational
shape? In answering these questions, we highlight the importance
of, sometimes hostile, outsider narratives about NICE, and the way
in which insiders engaged with these in constructing a place for the
Council. We will stress how the Institute had already created what
it regarded as important new processes for stakeholder participation.
It hence fashioned a particular vision of the Council – and
importantly of the kinds of questions that it would address – with
this in mind.

This chapter is in three parts. The first paints a picture of NICE at
the point where the Citizens Council idea began to develop, linking

understandings of the organisation with the challenge of putting words on paper about the precise shape of the Council. The second tracks back, piecing together what were the more specific sources for the idea of a council and making reference to the early discussions in NICE as its soon-to-be-host organisation, about the form it should take. In the third part, we examine what turned out to be a highly successful quest to find volunteers from among the population at large prepared to become citizens' councillors. We give an account of the process of recruiting them and we draw briefly on their own words, in interviews carried out between the induction and first meeting, as to why they had come forward. Finally, we offer a preliminary assessment of some of the features of the design choices that were made about the Council and some hints about how consequential these choices were to become.

Data sources are several. They include perusal of a range of documents, both those in the public domain and not; a round of interviews with senior staff in NICE carried out late in 2002; observation at meetings of the steering committee set up by NICE to have oversight of the process; and informal discussions, held over a two-year period, with the then full-time Citizens Council project manager. Despite the substantial degree of access this afforded, we faced one particular practical difficulty. Commissioned in the late summer of 2002 to carry out what was to be a two-year evaluation, the research team appeared on the scene a matter of just weeks before that November induction meeting. If we were to understand the origins of the Council we were going to have to track back, finding relevant documents and relying on memories where 'how it is now' inevitably coloured recollections of how it was then. Appendix 1 sets out key aspects of the research design, and Appendix 5 lists the main documentary sources that were consulted in the course of the study.

Narratives about NICE

NICE was still a fairly new organisation at the time that the Citizens Council emerged. It had begun work in the spring of 1999, having been first announced in a White Paper six months after Labour took office in 1997 (DH, 1997). Its aim was to deliver guidance on treatments to the health service in England and Wales in order to ensure equal access for all patients to the most clinically effective and (more controversially) cost-effective health technologies. It was one of a network of new regulatory bodies in health (Walshe, 2002), working at arm's length but responsible directly to the Secretary of State through the Department of Health. Over its first three years of existence, its activity programme had evolved from technology appraisals, dealing with specific drugs and devices, to include the development of national guidelines for whole conditions. Subsequently its work was to extend still further (see Appendix 4).

The remit of the Institute proved to be controversial in the eyes of many. When the Citizens Council was announced, the *British Medical Journal*, for example, pounced on a 'toothless tiger' accusation by the Patients' Association, linking it with the claim of one parliamentarian that the government was already hiding behind the 'fig leaf' of NICE to cover its funding decisions (Gulland, 2002). A cartoon portraying the Institute as the Prime Minister's puppet had already found its way onto the wall of the chair of NICE's office. It was clear, too, that each time the Institute issued draft or final guidance on a drug, the national press was going to take an interest and to seek divergent viewpoints. Academics have cast a critical eye over the political significance of the Institute (see, for example, The POWER Inquiry, 2006), often couching their assessments starkly in terms of 'rationing' (see Appleby and Coote, 2002; Ham and Robert, 2003). For those within the Institute, however, there were more immediate critics with whom to contend.

Among clinicians, the predominant fear early on was that NICE would mean the loss of the autonomy they had long enjoyed in relation to individual decisions concerning patient care and that was central to their understandings of professional identities. Clinical scepticism focused on a charge of 'cookbook medicine' (Sackett et al, 1996; Charlton and Miles, 1998), and on the Institute as serving a political purpose in controlling doctors. Charlton, pursuing this line, went on to conjure up the dire prediction that:

> ... doctors who disobey NICE recommendations will be harassed, humiliated, sacked or struck off the medical register. (Charlton, 2000: 30)

The pharmaceutical industry also portrayed NICE as a threat. The national and international row brought about by the very first drug appraisal dealing with the flu drug Relenza brought home just how deep the conflict could go. The industry already had to demonstrate safety, quality and efficacy to the Medicines Control Agency before it could launch a new drug on the market. NICE's remit regarding cost-effectiveness seemed to be adding a "fourth hurdle" (Gopal, 1999: 36).

The chair of Glaxo Wellcome, in a letter leaked to the *Sunday Telegraph*, wrote to the Secretary of State claiming that the work of NICE "called into question the suitability of the UK as a base for multinational pharmaceutical operations" (Gopal, 1999: 35). The *Financial Times*, having published rather similar sentiments in a letter from another chief executive officer, offered the sardonic leader comment that what appeared to have stunned the industry was that NICE "wanted evidence, not assumptions" (*Financial Times*, 4 October 1999).

Conflicts proliferated. 'NICE blight' came into common parlance as a term describing a situation where the NHS was seemingly unwilling to support the prescribing of a drug whose future was uncertain, thereby undermining the launch or the continuing sales of a medicine (Gopal, 2001). The concept lingered, particularly among those in NHS trusts who regularly reported to the local 'roadshows' which accompanied bimonthly NICE board meetings, that they found it difficult to make decisions about using a treatment once it was under NICE appraisal.

Organised patient groups, as we saw in Chapter One, were newly finding a voice and a place at the health policy table. Quennell (2001), interviewing some of those participating in early drug appraisals in the Institute, found that developments were "somewhat ad hoc". As one of her respondents put it:

> In the early days of NICE it was really chaotic, and they made lots of mistakes, both in terms of they hadn't thought, so they were inventing it as they went along.... And then what would happen is that they would just make an administrative cock-up with large consequences for somebody. (Quennell, 2001: 205)

Patient and carer representatives had taken the initiative in setting up an informal support group: Patients Involved in NICE (PIN). Subsequently the Institute itself established and funded a Patient Involvement Unit (PIU), with the responsibility of helping to identify appropriate organisations to consult on a particular topic, and seeking nominations from individuals and groups to join appraisal committees and review documents and processes. Later the remit extended to include the direct provision of forms of training and support for this activity.

The possibility that there would be multiple critics of the Institute had already found structural reflection in the creation of a Partners

Council. This is a 45-strong body appointed by the Secretary of State, with a statutory duty to meet once a year and to review the Annual Report. It provides an opportunity for stakeholders to express any concerns and to raise questions about directions of work and future plans. Patient and carer organisation representatives and representatives from the different professions constitute the two largest groupings, alongside those from the healthcare industries, NHS management and trades unions. Clearly, then, there were multiple arenas in which an interest would be likely to be taken in the fledgling Citizens Council.

What of understandings from within of the significance of NICE? Organisation members, Weick (1979: 243) reminds us, "construct, rearrange, single out and demolish" features of their surroundings. And in the doing of this, what begins to emerge is the creation of one or more organisational narratives, stories, that is, "that underlie the values and assumptions of an organisation and link the members into a group" (Polkinghorne, 1988: 162). Such narratives, variable in their coherence and in the degree to which they are shared, can be found in publicity documents, on websites and in the words of the organisational members themselves. Our initial round of interviews, carried out at the end of 2002, can be seen in this light. Located in a public sector setting, interviewees, not surprisingly, took themes from an official discourse of public policy, the White Paper, for example, that introduced NICE, and the subsequent consultation document that linked it more firmly to the quality improvement agenda in the NHS (DH, 1997, 1998). Their accounts refracted such themes through the histories of staff themselves and their prior experience and identities – particularly as clinicians and managers in the health service. What was also striking, however, at least among this group of most senior people involved in the Institute, was the degree to which their accounts echoed one another.

At least five interrelated discursive themes emerged from early interviews, providing interpretative resources for potential organisational narratives. First, the senior staff often distanced themselves from a tight link with the immediate elements of the Labour project. They constructed themselves and the Institute as connecting with a longer line of evidence-based endeavour, bringing order into a confusion of pre-existing local guidelines including those produced by the medical profession. One person explained:

> "There had been attempts at producing guidance from
> the Royal Colleges. But when they were assessed ... their

quality was found to be very variable. They [the guidelines] were also 'aspirational' – what we would like in an ideal world. So they were never fully implemented because it isn't a perfect world.... Often they were lobbying documents – such as 'we need more cardiologists!' And many of them were contradictory."

Holding the ring between such aspirants, bringing order into the multiple and chaotic initiatives of the past, and doing this through careful interrogations of evidence, were key elements of the internal meaning making in NICE. In this frame, the organisation's work could be positioned not as 'cookbook medicine' at all, but as a resource offering positive help to the busy clinician. "NICE is there to translate research into practice," said one director. Another added:

"All the areas we work in have some uncertainty associated with. NICE provides a fix for the NHS and for the people who use it at a particular point in time."

A second discursive theme invoked the notion of 'pioneering', doing what no one had done before, working in uncharted waters, and devising new solutions as they went along. Part of this had to do with how national guidance was being developed in association with stakeholders. "We are breaking new boundaries," said a director; "now patients, professionals and the public can work together to improve health care". For some participants, such a construction was linked both with a new kind of practice and with a return to the importance of what they saw as earlier NHS ideals – what the Institute was doing was "putting the 'national' back into the national health service".

Third, 'priority setting' replaced 'rationing' in the lexicon of the Institute. "Rationing," objected one director, "conjures up World War Two and an indiscriminate allocation of so much resources to each person, whereas prioritisation means actively considering what we are able to commit and making decisions within that". There was the added point that NICE guidance was authoritative, in its expert and multifaceted review of available evidence, but it remained guidance. Local health authorities and individual clinicians still took the decision on the specific locality and case (see Appendix 4).

Fourth, the fact that all this inevitably meant working in the spotlight was both clearly identified and recognised in these accounts. It was also framed in a way that positively welcomed engagement with critics, and celebrated this as part of the perceived robustness of a new and improved evidence assessment process that was the key feature of the Institute. Interviewees constructed their audience as much more all-encompassing than the immediate critics and potential local users of guidance. They proudly pointed out that the formal pronouncements on drugs from NICE were attracting widespread international attention.

Fifth, in this environment of continuing controversy, where counter-narratives questioned the legitimacy of the organisation, participants construed themselves as people who were constantly listening, balancing, being 'independent' and acting with integrity. There was a real need, one person explained, to establish credibility and authority:

> "It isn't enough to have a formal role and government backing. That doesn't create trust – it only comes with time and credibility."

Being able to enter into the discourses of their critics, being able, reflectively for example, to deploy the 'fig leaf' accusation and publicly to acknowledge the meanings conveyed by terms like 'NICE blight' could serve to anticipate and to some extent to disarm potential critics.

The ways in which these senior members of the Institute constructed accounts of the organisation were bound up with some core practices defining this still newly emerging community. Routines and procedures put into practice aimed to be *inclusive* of all those with a relevant interest in the issue; to be *open* to new ideas and open also in making both plans and ways of working transparent; and to be *revisable*. Senior staff repeatedly stressed how important it was to be flexible and they were keen to hear new ideas as to how to carry out their remit better. Giving time to make a large volume of material freely available on the website and allocating resources to ensure that it stayed up to date was one feature. Another was the decision to appoint a director of communications with a place on the main board. Holding regular 'roadshows' at venues around the country, inviting comment and criticism at these and also bringing critics in for discussion, and referring to policies not as fixed tests but as 'living documents', subject to routine revision, were still others. Such practices could serve to mollify critics, although they did not always do so.

Commitments to openness and inclusivity were especially visible in the routines that were established for mainstream activity. Box 3.1 sets out the way of working for the appraisal programme as they were put on paper in 2003. Two things are striking about the textual representation of this procedure (designed to be completed within a target period in each case of some 62 weeks). The first is its striving towards inclusiveness of the many stakeholder interests, the second is its staged character, allowing for multiple points of dialogue with different communities of interest.

In principle, this documentation imagines different kinds of knowledge coming into play from the start. Scientific and technical knowledge is gathered together by a team from an academic centre. Knowledge 'with an interest' is represented by the pharmaceutical companies, suppliers and manufacturers, who themselves fund trials and whose evidence is part of the material to be assessed. Challenge to both of these is possible from organised patient groups, who may have initiated research, or whose research staff may propose different overall assessments of the assembled material. These groups also consult their members who live with the condition, and thus bring experiential knowledge into the frame. Further challenges can also come from the experience of practising clinicians and from the perspectives of health service managers, who have to balance the implications of implementing a recommendation for one intervention against the funds foregone for the implementation of another. The stages where drafts and then final recommendations are made public serve to catapult the issue into a wider public arena. Interviewees highlighted how the draft recommendation consultation (point 7) was often 'misunderstood' or even seemingly at times exploited by external stakeholders to stimulate public reaction.

Box 3.1: Steps in the appraisal process

1. Referral to NICE from the Department of Health/National Assembly for Wales.
2. Internal review to identify stakeholder organisations that need to be consulted – including patient/carer organisations, healthcare professions and manufacturers.
3. Consultation with stakeholders on the scope of the appraisal – including the coverage of patient groups and the sources of evidence.
4. Academic centre commissioned to produce an independent review of published evidence – the assessment report.
5. Appraisal committee meets to consider the assessment report and to take verbal and written evidence from stakeholders.
6. Preliminary recommendation prepared based on all evidence received thus far – the appraisal consultation document.

7. Document sent out for a four-week consultation; also posted on the website.
8. Appraisal committee meets again to consider feedback and prepare final recommendation.
9. This document, the final appraisal determination, is posted on the website for information.
10. Stakeholder organisations are offered a limited period in which to appeal.
11. An Appeal Panel hears any appeals and NICE makes amendments or resubmits it to the independent committee to look again at the evidence and recommendations prior to guidance being issued.
12. Guidance is issued to the NHS.

Source: NICE (2003: 10-11)

The key question for this chapter is just how an organisation with these accounting frames and core practices would deal with the Citizens Council idea. On the one hand, a council would certainly seem to fit with the open and inclusive ethos. If ways had already been found for including 'the public in particular' in developing guidance, ways of including 'the public in general' might well appear as a natural next step. On the other hand, there was a very real issue of how to integrate views from the public into the kind of process set out in Box 3.1. In practice, as the next section will show, what the Institute did was to position the Citizens Council at one remove from the daily business of devising guidance, and to adopt what was in effect a modified citizens' jury model for its design.

Assimilating and activating the Council project

The announcement in the government's NHS Plan in the summer of 2000 that there would be a Citizens Council in NICE (DH, 2000) did not come out of the blue for members of the Institute. Senior figures were already in frequent contact with officials and ministers. How exactly did the idea for a Citizens Council emerge? No one was prepared to name an exact time, a single person or a specific place. However, interviewees pointed to the importance of involvement in the government's Modernisation Action Teams that had preceded the Plan, and to the interest in the issue both from the Prime Minister's advisory unit in Downing Street and from the new Strategy Unit in the Department of Health.

A first Institute document, tentatively setting out a model for the

Council, was dated three months after the NHS Plan was published. Produced by the chair of NICE, it proposed the Citizens Council as a standing committee of the board, with the aim:

> ... to consider, at the request of the Board of the National Institute for Clinical Excellence, matters requiring a broad-based general view so as to assist the Institute in the performance of its functions. (NICE draft policy document, October 2000: App 5)

The document went on to outline a council of 30 members, representative of the public in terms of gender, ethnicity, socioeconomic status and age. At this point, it was to meet three times a year, and it was to be chaired by the chair of the Institute himself.

The chief executive and the chair met several times with staff at the Strategy Unit on the matter and a second document was drawn up by Professor Chris Ham, a key figure at that time in the Unit, and addressed to the Chief Medical Officer for comment. This now offered a more detailed rationale for the notion of a 'broad-based view', stressing the need to explore the value judgements surrounding the key activities of NICE:

> Experience of priority setting, both in the UK and other countries, has highlighted the fact that decisions on the funding of health technologies and pathways of care cannot invariably be resolved by scientific evidence and expert opinion. Of course, evidence from clinical trials and cost-effectiveness studies, and the views of clinicians and economists, play an important part in informing decision making. Priority setting, however, often involves making value judgements about the use of resources and their allocation between competing claims. These value judgements may apply both to individual technologies and to decisions about the relative priority to be given to different technologies or treatment programmes. (DH, Strategy Unit, 2001: App 5)

The memorandum went on to consider practicalities of how the Council might operate. Taking its standing committee character and a three-year term of office as given, the regular retirement of perhaps one third, would mean "combining a degree of consistency with an element of freshness" (ibid). The number 30 was endorsed on the grounds that "the Council needs to be small enough to work efficiently and big enough to reflect different points of view" (ibid). Various recruitment models were reviewed. Members could be appointed or randomly selected from electoral registers ensuring a cross-section of social groups. Whatever the method, the main issue was that the process must be seen to be fair and Council members should reflect the society from which they were drawn. The memorandum also came down in favour of members being *new* to the issues, not health professionals or employees of healthcare industries and not people involved in patient groups. Three further parameters were set. The Council should meet in public. There should be "a small permanent staff to provide administrative and other support" (ibid), and a dedicated additional budget. Joint working between the Strategy Unit and the top tier of NICE had thus set out key contours for the Citizens Council.

The idea of operating at one remove from the appraisals work, and of seeking underlying value judgements, was positioned prominently in what was referred to as the final operating model for the Council, set out in a revision to a working document in April 2002 by the chair. The questions to be asked "would be general in nature, relating to social, ethical or moral questions"(DH, Strategy Unit, 2001: App 5). The unmentioned background to this decision was the Institute's resistance to initial departmental pressure to have the Council debate its individual appraisals. Internally, it was felt that NICE was still too tender in years and status to cope with such a proposal. There had been mention, however, of the possibility that Citizens Council members themselves might join members of the appraisals and guidelines committees in generating suitable topics.

Box 3.2: Question for the first Citizens Council meeting

What should NICE take into account when making decisions about clinical need?

There are three key elements that NICE would like the Citizens Council to consider specifically. These are:

13. The most important features of diseases, or conditions, that should be taken into account when deciding clinical need.
14. The most important features of patients, rather than their condition, that should be taken into account.

15. The weight the Institute should give to the views of each of the various groups of stakeholders (consultees) in deciding clinical need.

Box 3.2 lays out the question that emerged from this focus on value judgements and that was presented to the Citizens Council at its first meeting in November 2002. In one sense, this formulation went directly to the heart of the dilemmas in the Institute's formal remit – to make decisions on the clinical effectiveness but also on the cost-effectiveness of interventions. If the clinical effectiveness of an intervention could be proven, what other criteria should come into play? What kind of reasoning supported other criteria? How much would this reasoning be likely to attract public support? Those who had had experience of the appraisal process (Box 3.1) were acutely aware of the uncertainties that could surround clinical data. They had experience of ways that efforts at influence and lobbying could be brought to bear. Ultimately, judgements had to come into play, and the idea of finding a more transparent and defensible framework to use at this point in the process was attractive. The exact wording of the clinical need question, as interviewees recalled, had been a result of much discussion and debate. There had been two topic-setting workshops where senior staff and programme directors had engaged in vigorous debate. But did 'clinical need' set out in this way give the Citizens Council a viable task to do and one that would make sense to them? Our micro-investigation set out in Chapter Four provides an opportunity to consider at close quarters just what happened.

A framework was now firmly in place, but there were still myriad issues to confront before those 30 people made their way to that London hotel early in November 2002. After recruitment delays, the project manager came into post in April 2002. She needed to develop and oversee a recruitment process for the citizens, and to bring the Institute's communications team into the picture in order to attend to the publicity that all felt certain the Council would attract. Working with a newly formed in-house steering committee, she needed to design and finalise a shape for the Council meetings. Only when this was done, would it be possible to begin to contact potential witnesses and secure a place in no doubt already full diaries. The project manager reviewed different models for citizen participation, but, by this time, the operating model was in its third draft and it was already 21 months since the formal announcement in the NHS Plan. To encompass reflection on alternatives at this point ran the risk of going backwards instead of forward.

Work proceeded apace. Separate tenders were drawn up for recruitment and facilitation of the Council, but, in the event, the company who bid successfully for the recruitment was invited to re-tender also for the facilitation contract. Vision 21 was a small social research company with a strong background in running citizens' juries. It was also, as a member of the selection panel put it, "spot on in terms of their complete grasp of what we wanted to do". NEXUS, a small media relations company with whom the Institute had worked before, was commissioned to help with publicity and provide the new Council members with the skills they would need for an anticipated media onslaught. The operating model had not considered that the Council members would need an induction, but the project manager's early literature search persuaded her of the necessity for this, and it also featured in Vision 21's proposals. It was duly incorporated. Last but not least was settling the actual design of the Council meetings. Vision 21 joined the steering committee in fusing their previous experience with the requirements of the project, and over a series of meetings a final pattern emerged. There was much urgency in all of this. If a range and balance of top class 'expert witnesses' were to be recruited for information giving at a first meeting before the end of the year, they needed to be contacted almost immediately.

Box 3.3: The initial design of the Citizens Council

Membership – 30 people, without any clinical affiliation or other link with the NHS and its industries.

Terms and conditions – appointment for up to three years, with regular replacement of 10 to ensure 'freshness'; payment of £150 per session; all travel and accommodation to be reimbursed.

Meetings – for around three days over a weekend, twice a year.

Format – citizens' jury style, with witness sessions and review at the core, and facilitated by a group external to the Institute.

Topic – to discuss questions of values, which would be devised and agreed by the steering committee in NICE.

Output – a report drawn up by facilitators, and presented by the Citizens Council committee to the board.

By way of summary, Box 3.3 brings together the key elements of the final design for the Council as these had been crystallised in the operating model. The total group was to number 30. All expenses for meetings at venues across the country were to be covered and the work was also to attract a fee. Mindful of the need not to 'capture' or 'contaminate' members, a 'retirement' plan had been devised. The Council resembled citizens' juries in its format, although as a standing body it might be seen more as a panel. The notion of a values question, which we have already begun to examine, was firmly in place. Responsibility for how results would be fed back into the Institute was placed in the hands of the chief executive. Before turning to some further comments on this set of decisions, we need to examine one further vitally important issue. Just who were the citizens on the Citizens Council? And why did they choose to take part?

Enter the citizens

From the beginning, NICE had prioritised social inclusion as a key characteristic of the Citizens Council. The operating model had specified a Council representative of the population in terms of gender, social class, ethnicity, age, geography and disability. In this NICE was strongly supported by Vision 21; the agency had its own political commitment to bringing the voices of 'hard-to-reach' groups into the policy arena. Recruitment for the Citizens Council proved a resounding success, in terms of the sheer volume of initial responses and the diversity of the eventual members. How was this achieved?

Advertisements were placed in regional and national media (including eight national and 70 local newspapers), and posters were sent out to GP surgeries and Citizens' Advice Bureaux. The advertisement (Box 3.4), under the banner 'Have your say in the NHS', certainly produced a good response, although it also perhaps raised unrealistic expectations about the range of issues that the Council would be able to address. Vision 21, drawing on their networks in working with hard-to-reach groups and their own grass-roots database, contacted the minority ethnic press, and mounted an e-mail campaign. They used 190 different networks, some targeting specific groups, such as the UK Youth Parliament. The advertisement in Wales went out in Welsh. NEXUS drafted press releases and organised editorial coverage. NICE played its part. The chief executive went on Breakfast TV and the chair was interviewed

Box 3.4: Advertisement for Citizens Council members

on Radio 4's *Today* programme. The results of all this activity were truly impressive. A stunning 35,000 expressions of interest flowed in. Application forms were sent out. They were kept simple, and there were large print and Braille versions, as well as tape-recorded and British Sign Language versions.

In all, just under 4,500 completed application forms were received: "It was really encouraging to get that number – people were so glad, so enthusiastic…. It made you realise you were working on something so important to the public," said a staff member of Vision 21. The agency coped with the task of producing a symbolically representative Council of 30 by first creating a bank of 350 names, stratified demographically according to the latest Office for National Statistics data. Then, through a process of telephone calls, and weeding out and matching up different combinations, they arrived at a group that not only mirrored the major demographic groups, but also provided a good range of experience and attitudes (see Davies et al, 2005: 47-8,180). Of the 30 members, 15 were women and 15 men. Ages ranged from 18 to 76. From 'housewife' to electrician, from retired civil servant to retail clerk, from builder to pilot, from make-up artist to printer, from security officer to teacher: Council members reflected a broad spectrum of working backgrounds, gathered from all corners of England and Wales (NICE press release, 8 November 2002). The full list of members of the original Citizens Council, as set out in this document, is shown in Appendix 2.

Why had the citizens wanted to be there in the first place? Our interviews were conducted by telephone in the short time between the induction meeting at the start of the month and the first full meeting of the Council, held in Salford on the weekend of 21 November 2002. They suggested three ways in which at that point they were making sense of the situation and justifying their decisions to become involved. First, responding directly perhaps to the framing in the advertisement for Council members, was the notion that 'people like me should have a say' in the running of public services. As one person explained:

> "These big public bodies seem to ... be run very much ... I won't say a closed shop exactly, that's probably the wrong wording to use, but they can be very remote and very distant from the general public. With it being a public service, I think the public should be slightly more involved in it. I realise that there are some decisions that have got to be taken by managers and all the rest of it, but I think some things could be ... more open to discussion, put it that way." (Martin)

Second, there were accounts that seemed to entail a sense of citizenship identity and public duty. Neither of these terms was employed directly. Wanting to "make a contribution", to "do something worthwhile", to "make a difference", to "benefit the future of our children" and to "put something back", were some of the phrases commonly used. Improving the NHS was a big factor here, again echoing that line in the advertisement that had first drawn their attention to the possibility of joining the Council:

> "We've got some difficult things to ... crack in the coming years, such as ... an ageing population and just the old classic expectations against a not unlimited budget.... I want to improve things and get an NHS that we, as a nation, are proud of.... We've got problems, people are getting better treatment in other countries, we want to be the leading

edge and the best in the provision of health services."
(Guy)

If belief in the importance of public involvement and a desire to help improve the NHS were two key ways of initially constructing a new subject position as Citizens Council member, a third came in the shape of personal growth and fulfilment. One person, wrapping this together with improving the NHS, asked:

> "What am I hoping to achieve? Well to ... have an experience ... on a committee or council like this; to, you know, grow myself as a person who can, you know, enter a discussion and put something positive in to it. For my own personal growth and for having an input in to an institution that affects everybody at some time in their life." (Jim)

Others also talked of "stretching" themselves. It was going to be "a way of getting my brain back into gear". It would be "a knowledge adventure ... to learn more and get involved with different organisations which represent the public, and different communities". People made reference to the varied life experiences they felt they could bring to bear. They also frequently referred to a sense of being "privileged" to have been selected. But there was also considerable uncertainty and anxiety, since they just did not know what to expect:

> "I was very, very nervous about how it was all going to go. I was very nervous about meeting everyone and sticking out like a sore thumb really. I had the impression that everyone was going to be quite professional and, you know, know all they were going to do, and I was going to be sat in the background, like, oh my God, what am I doing this for?" (Rachael)

Notable by its absence from almost all of the accounts, was explicit reference to the work of NICE, its specific role in relation to the NHS and the controversies that have been outlined earlier in the chapter. The significance of this will become apparent in the chapters that follow. For now, however, and building on the material in Part I of this book, what might be concluded at this point about some of the challenges that the design would be likely to produce?

Conclusion

Social institutions, as we emphasised at the outset, are never created totally anew. They reflect the experience of their creators, the context in which those people find themselves and the complex ways in which both are refracted through the sense-making activity and narratives of key participants. This chapter has aimed to put flesh on this proposition, highlighting the way in which design decisions arose from the specific circumstances of the time, and the struggle to create solutions that would be workable for the Institute in the light of its understandings of its role and the commitments that had arisen from this.

Undoubtedly, the citizens' jury model was in the minds of the early architects of the Citizens Council. We saw in Chapter One how central this model was to new forms of citizen participation in local government and the NHS, and in Chapter Two how early evaluations put juries in a particularly positive light. Some of those involved with the 1990s' citizens' juries were now close to the centre of government. One of the directors of the Institute confirmed not only that examples of juries constituted the majority of cases they found, but also that these were particularly attractive in the way they used members of the public, accessed witnesses and were deliberative. The fact that Vision 21 had had direct experience of setting up and running citizens' juries and of recruiting members from hard-to-reach groups reflected and reinforced this focus on the jury model.

Several modifications occurred. The jury was larger than usual, 30 people instead of the more usual 12 or so, and it had some permanency. Two points stand out here. First, it was simply not open to the Institute to use the conventional one-off jury. The commitment in the NHS Plan pointed quite clearly to something that would bring the public into the Institute in a more enduring way. And it did not take much reflection to see that recruiting a new jury each time on a national scale would be prohibitively resource consuming. Second, the Institute already had a fairly complex, and in some ways still novel, set of participative and consultative processes. Integrating 'the public' into this process was not straightforward and the suggestion was resisted. From these two commitments flowed the twin ideas of creating a *standing* council and keeping it *at one remove* from the day-to-day decision making. And other implications started to emerge. To end the chapter, we can briefly explore just three of these.

First, *there is the question of the question*. Citizens' juries in the main are asked fairly straightforward questions, ones that are often of direct personal interest. They have been used, as one reviewer put it, for "specific, practical planning issues, within a very narrowly defined remit" (Pickard, 1998: 241). NICE, as the early documentation has revealed, aimed to formulate more of a 'meta-'question – to tap the values that might inform and underpin the questions it was already facing about the clinical and cost-effectiveness of a particular intervention. One member of the Vision 21 team, recalling first contact with the Institute, remembered feeling puzzled on this score. The Institute seemed to be "very, very clear" about the number of members and levels of pay, for example, but not about what they were going to discuss. "With other citizens' juries, they know what they want to know" (Vision 21 team member). In what follows, again and again, we will see a struggle with the question on the part of all participants. It was not perhaps that the Institute did not know what it wanted to know. It was more that whether what it wanted to know was knowable and could be successfully elicited by means of a jury approach.

Second, *there is the nature of the relationship between the host and the Council.* The steering committee had shown a strong desire not to influence the Council. There had been concern from the outset in the documentation about keeping the Council fresh (the stress on the regular retirement policy, for example) and avoiding the potential of capture by the host. Recruitment and facilitation work had been outsourced. The chair, introducing himself and the Institute at the induction, and again at the first meeting, stressed the importance of the Council's independence, and joked "we don't want to contaminate you". The operating model did not dwell at all on the issue of just how much the citizens would need to understand the purposes and processes of the organisation they were being asked to help. A brief initial introduction to the work of NICE and presentations from the three programme directors at the first meeting served as orientation. We will see that thinking later shifted – fear of capture was replaced by a recognition of the need to give the citizens much more of a sense, for example, of what it was that the Institute's appraisal process entailed.

Third, *there is the issue of the Council output and its impact.* In the case of a citizens' jury commissioned by a local authority, there is an expectation of a reasonably clear decision on a topic known to be controversial. This decision is fed back to and debated by a body accountable to the local electorate, a body that is usually debating in public. Intense media interest often aids the transparency of the process. The argument usually is that the jury output, while it can guide decisions and add more information (what a group of the public would think if exposed to information and opportunities for debate), it cannot in itself be definitive – elected representatives must decide. Where the host is an organisation, however, and one of the complexity of NICE, there are no easy answers to the question of exactly when and where 'the join' takes place. The operating model envisaged a report to the board and allocated responsibility to the chief executive for disseminating the Council's advice within the Institute. Interviewees spoke in broad terms of the output being "helpful". Just what a report giving "a broad-based general view" would look like and how it would "assist" the Institute in the performance of its "functions" (phrases used in the first internal document on the Council), remained unspecified as the first meeting loomed. For a really alert observer, a description of the Council as "a backdrop of public opinion against which we and the independent groups that advise us can make their recommendations" (NICE press release, 19 August 2002), might have rung some warning bells.

To read this account as setting out matters that "could have been resolved" is to oversimplify. There was an important sense in which the Institute was breaking new ground in trying to fashion a rather different kind of jury, seeking to utilise it in the context of an organisation with cross-cutting participatory processes already in place. Interwoven with the questions being raised here were deeper ones – to do with just what 'the public' could be asked to do and how, and whether the hopes that are pinned particularly on deliberative modes of participation are both justifiable and realisable. All of these questions will come to the fore as the following chapters unfold.

FOUR

Doing deliberation: the first Citizens Council meeting

It was inevitable that the Institute's operating model would construct 'the citizen' and 'deliberation' in particular ways and would rely on a mix of explicit, implicit and sometimes contradictory assumptions and premises that would only come into sharper focus once the Council had met. This chapter thus explores what occurred as the Citizens Council migrated from an in-house organisational plan to an actual embodied event, in other words, as the meso-level gave way to the micro-level. What consequences flowed from the attempt to implement the model? Would the hopes and ambitions of the advocates of the ideal of deliberative participation be realised? Would the positive and negative experiences reported in accounts of local one-off citizens' juries be reproduced in a national high-profile standing council?

This chapter – the first of three drawing on transcripts of video records of the events, ethnographic observations and quantitative analyses – provides a detailed account of the first meeting, held at a hotel in Salford late in November 2002, and the nature of the challenges it posed. The next chapter will then go on to explore changes to the design for later meetings and their impact. Both chapters link the analysis to the question that has already been explored in some detail in the empirical research on more conventional forms of citizens' juries, of what practical lessons can be drawn. Thus far, however, there have been very few studies that might be described as ethnographies of democratic deliberation. This study is the first description of a deliberative forum based on a data corpus made up from videotaped records of the series of events (28,857 lines of transcript in the case of the first meeting alone).

The first section describes the balance of activities that made up the Salford meeting. The second section goes on to look at the process of becoming informed. What sense did the members of the Council make of the material they were given? What stance did they take in relation to the expert witnesses and in what sense were discussions informed by the material presented by witnesses? In the third section, the evidence for deliberation, dialogue, debate and discussion is examined. Did deliberation in the senses described in the early parts of Chapter Two actually occur? The fourth section moves to the process of reaching conclusions for a report. The final section considers a further key component of a deliberative forum: inclusiveness. Did some voices dominate? Were some excluded altogether? For the first Citizens Council meeting some of these key dimensions of deliberation proved very challenging and the chapter will explore why this was so.

What does a Citizens Council do?

In answering this question, NICE and Vision 21, the facilitators contracted to run the event, were guided by many of the settled practices characteristic of citizens' juries reviewed in Part I. The NICE Citizens Council in the course of a three-day residential event would debate a question: 'What should NICE take into account when making decisions about clinical need?'. (See Box 3.2 in Chapter Three for the full wording.) To make sure that citizens were sufficiently informed, expert witnesses would be called to give evidence and citizens would have the chance to question and interrogate these witnesses. Citizens would work in small groups on sub-tasks and themes and in plenary sessions with the whole Council to mull over this evidence and to reach conclusions. The report would be written by the facilitators but checked with the citizens to ensure it was a faithful record of the decisions made.

Citizens' juries vary in how much control the citizens can exert over the process. How much would be 'up to them' in this case? Very little. The witnesses had been pre-selected by NICE and Vision 21; the question was set in advance and was not pre-circulated to the councillors before the event started. The organisers also set the timetable for each day. There was, in fact, a 'quiet revolution' at the beginning of the second day and the councillors asked for a closed session without the facilitators, the research team, the NICE project manager or the Institute's communications team. We cannot know what was discussed in this session but the result was that the Council expressed unhappiness with how the event was proceeding, particularly with the wording of the question, although they decided to continue with the organisational plan.

During most sessions the Council sat in boardroom style. Each person's name was visible on a card in front of them and each had an individual microphone. When they wished to speak or ask a question they turned their name card on one side as a signal to the facilitator (sitting at the 'high table' on one side of the square), and when called to speak switched on their microphone. They learned to help one another, leaning over to switch on the microphone for visually impaired colleagues, or for someone who had forgotten to do this. For most of the citizen councillors this was very unfamiliar territory, although some did have experience of committee work and participation in large assemblies. These procedural aspects of working together as a Council fairly quickly became habits, however, and remained unchanged in subsequent meetings.

The facilitation team consisted of five members. There were two lead facilitators (one male and one female) who chaired most of the plenary sessions and many of the small groups, and two female members who acted as the 'councillors' friends', managing the practical organisation of the meeting, supporting citizens with disabilities, acting as note takers for the final report and chairing some small groups. The final member of the team was an ex-NHS chief executive who also facilitated some of the plenary sessions but whose main role was described as the 'logic observer'. In citizens' juries, 'logic observers' are deployed to follow the unfolding reasoning of the jury and to keep it on track (Stewart et al, 1994). In this instance, however, the term had a rather different connotation. The logic observer was described as a 'living dictionary', his role being to answer any factual queries on the workings of the health service. The NICE project manager was also present, together with a two-man communications team from NEXUS contracted to manage media interest. In the event, there was very little media interest at this meeting or at subsequent ones; a few newspaper reporters mostly from regional papers occasionally sat in on sessions. Most plenary and witness sessions were open to the general public as well as the press, and a few people were there to watch the proceedings, while the small groups were closed to the press and the public. Finally, present throughout were three (and sometimes four) members of the research team as observers, and the three-man film crew recording the event.

The core activities of the NICE Citizens Council (witness presentations, questions to witnesses, small group work, review sessions and process talk) are described in more detail in Box 4.1, while Figure 4.1 indicates the balance among these activities that defined the tone and tenor of the meeting. Members of the Council spent most of their time in plenary sessions, and about a quarter of the time working in small groups. Time was fairly equally split between sessions designed to inform and educate about the topic (the witness and questions to witnesses sessions), and those discussing the evidence (small group and review sessions). Clearly the balance set between acquiring information on the one hand and debate and discussion on the other would have a major impact on the flavour and nature of the Council.

The deliberative ideal involves citizens coming together to reflect on and discuss an often complex and controversial public issue. For this, participants need background information and exposure to a whole gamut of competing views. A study of early citizens' juries in the UK (Coote and Lenaghan, 1997) opened up the tricky question of balance, indicating how contentious the issue of the right amount of information can be. While they report a feeling among the jurors that they would have liked more information and more time with witnesses, the authors themselves recommended only four witnesses a day with a maximum of 45 minutes each, as "too many perspectives can confuse rather than illuminate the issues" (Coote and Lenaghan, 1997: 80). In this first meeting of the NICE Citizens Council the balance seemed rather weighted towards acquiring information. A lot was to depend, however, on the actual context and experience of the different kinds of sessions and these aspects will be examined throughout the rest of this chapter.

Figure 4.1: Proportion of activities in the first Citizens Council meeting

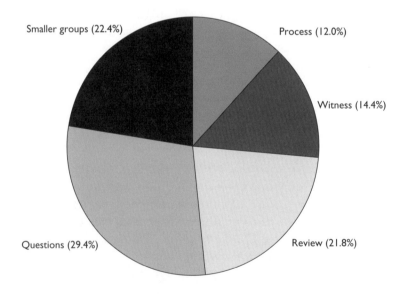

Smaller groups (22.4%)

Process (12.0%)

Witness (14.4%)

Questions (29.4%)

Review (21.8%)

Box 4.1: Activities in the first Citizens Council meeting

Witness presentations: the Council listened to presentations from 12 witnesses over the three days. These witnesses developed different perspectives on clinical need from a variety of expert perspectives and included, for example, a health economist and former NHS finance director, the manager of a carer's organisation, a former NHS chief executive and the medical director of the Association of British Pharmaceutical Industries. Other external speakers included representatives from NICE, for example, the chair of the board who introduced the question and explained the background. Witness presentations followed a relatively standard format – the witness spoke for between 20-40 minutes, usually without interruption, in lecture mode using an overhead projector or PowerPoint display. There was only one exception to this format – one expert conducted an exercise with the members of the Council using a case history of a real patient to explore the difference between values-based and evidence-based medicine.

Questions to witnesses: the question and answer sessions which followed each witness presentation normally lasted about 25-30 minutes and were tightly chaired by a facilitator.

Small group work: Council members were frequently split into small groups where they worked on tasks such as formulating questions to witnesses and working through case studies aimed at helping them to focus on clinical need. The facilitators set aside time in the small group sessions early in the meeting, for example, for the members of the Council to negotiate and discuss the points they wanted to follow up with each witness and to sketch out the questions they wished to address to them. The groups varied in size and composition ranging from two groups of 15 to three groups of 10. In this meeting all small groups were facilitated.

Review sessions: at strategic points (for example, at the end of each day and after a period of small group work) the facilitators provided an opportunity for the Council to review progress. Typically these plenary sessions focused on evaluating and recording the evidence presented by the witnesses. Facilitators worked with a flip chart and members of the Council were encouraged to call out points to record, written on the charts by a second facilitator or a Council member.

Process: a significant proportion of the meeting was spent in procedural talk. Procedural talk includes the interaction necessary to organise the meeting, discussion about the task itself that often occurred when the members of the Council were trying to work out what they should be doing or were unhappy about procedures.

Becoming informed

In a perfect world, the process of acquiring information through the questioning of expert witnesses would be straightforward. All the expert witnesses would be clear, accessible and coherent. The topic, too, although possibly opaque initially, would become clear and straightforward. The members of the Council would demonstrate a growing grasp of the issues, be empowered to ask highly pertinent questions, and all the participants would stay 'on message' all of the time. As Chapter Two noted, actual deliberation is likely to be very different from imagined deliberation and the process of becoming informed in fact throws up a number of dilemmas, some perilous to the very enterprise itself.

As a first exercise in simple quantification and to yield some indication of the 'health' of the information-giving process in the first Citizens Council meeting, all the questions members of the Council put to witnesses were examined. The nature of these questions should begin to indicate how far the expert witness sessions were fit for purpose and whether the topic of clinical need and the issues it raised were clear. Instances of 'focused questions' were thus coded and counted. A question was coded as focused if it met the following criteria. It was relevant (either implicitly or explicitly) both to the material presented by the witness, and it was relevant to the question set by NICE which was the main business of the Council. In technical terms, questions needed to demonstrate global topical relevance (van Dijk, 1980) in two senses – by reference to the topics set up by the witness and to the larger segment of the overall topic for the meeting. Focused questions could be evaluative or factual in nature. They might, for example, be short requests for more information, or they might be much longer interventions that argue for, or demonstrate, the speaker's own perspective on the issue as well as asking a question.

Extract 1 gives an example of a focused question taken from the third day of the meeting. The question is addressed to an expert witness who was the manager of a charity. This extract suggests a positive picture. A Citizens councillor is engaging here with an issue and working with a witness to find out the information she needs. Her question goes to the heart of the argument made by this witness, confirms her reading of his perspective and is clearly linked to the question of clinical need.

Extract 1

Cindy: "Hiya. We have to produce a report at the end of these three days to say what things we think NICE should take into account in making decisions about clinical need. And basically, I don't want to summarise what you've said, but are you saying that, um, the carer's view should really be taken and given a lot more emphasis, um, into deciding clinical need?"

Charity manager: "I think that yes, at the moment, the legislation in terms of planning for discharge, for instance, says that anybody who is intending to provide care can have an assessment, a carer's assessment, which is looking at their particular needs. And what we're basically saying is that that should be as soon as somebody is admitted to hospital, for instance. I'm using the sort of acute sector as an example. But then the question that should be asked: 'is there somebody who's been involved in their care, or is likely to be involved in their care, and if so what is going to be the situation?'. And if that's the reality, then they should be involved in that situation."

Cindy: "They should just be given a lot more weight in the power of decision?"

Moments such as this were rare in this first meeting. Only 28% of all the questions put to expert witnesses could be described as focused and many of these were simple requests for factual information. In general, the councillors reported that they experienced these question sessions as directionless and confusing. Indeed their disappointment with how things were going was part of the motive for their 'quiet revolution' on the second day, described above.

If there were so few focused questions, what was happening? Large numbers of questions picked up on points made by expert witnesses. They showed curiosity about aspects of the witnesses' working lives, but had no discernible relevance to the topic of clinical need. Quite a number of what could be called 'hobby horse' questions were posed. These were questions which were usually highly positioned (showing the speaker's own point of view), but with no relevance or engagement with the expert witness's actual presentation, and mixed, but usually low, relevance to the overarching question set for the Council. One of the members of the Council, for example, had a strongly held view that the NHS would be improved if matrons were reintroduced into hospitals, and he asked several witnesses about their own views on this matter. Another member of the Council was very much in favour of complementary medicine. In Extract 2, a question on this topic is being posed to one of the expert witnesses. It is clear from his response that this witness was at something of a loss and did not feel he was the right person to address this topic.

Extract 2

Fred: "Yes, my question to you is what research have you done into alternative medicines and drugs?"

NHS manager: "Can you repeat that, I am sorry?"

Fred: "Alternative medicine, yes?"

NHS manager: "Yes?"

Fred: "And drugs. What research, if any, has been done and the cost of it?"

NHS manager: "There is not as much, there is not a lot of research, I am not an expert on this...."

Were some types of witnesses or presentation styles more useful than others? The patterns for each witness were examined and there were few major differences. The witness who attracted the highest ratio of focused to other kinds of questions was a nurse/midwife who covered issues to do with cultural specificity. Council members engaged with this topic, and here their interest in her material coincided with the issue of clinical need. The most influential witness overall, as measured by the amount of times her points were cited and quoted in subsequent review sessions, was an expert patient witness. She was controversial, had a very clear investment, raised a concrete pro-and-con type of issue, developed a narrative and included a range of memorable anecdotes that the Citizens councillors could come back to in their reviews. There was also a strong emotional identification with her and her story. She was "useful", as one citizen put it, "as a first-hand person experiencing clinical need from her own viewpoint". There was little evidence, however, of participants tying their recollections specifically to the questions set.

Why were there not more focused questions? It may be that citizens' juries and deliberative assemblies are always somewhat circuitous; few studies thus far, however, have been able to employ the recording techniques that would pick this up. In this instance, investigations of the later Citizens Council meetings, and remarks from councillors later in the process, confirmed that there was a particular problem in the first meeting. It became evident that the question set by the Institute on clinical need was not sufficiently clear. Too many complex issues were pulled together under one umbrella; the question was phrased in an obscure and puzzling manner and was not concrete enough. The social value dimension of the question was difficult to disentangle, since the subsidiary questions (see Box 3.2, 'important features of diseases...'; 'important features of patients...') looked as though they demanded factual answers.

With hindsight it became obvious that the terminology ('clinical need') was too embedded in the discursive world of NICE rather than the life world of the public. Crucially, the members of the Council found it difficult to remember the question, or any definition of clinical need, from one session to the next. They therefore found it exceedingly hard to decide what information was necessary for them to make recommendations, and how the witnesses might help them. The problem was compounded because, due to anticipated media and lobby group interest, the Council was not given the question in advance of the meeting. Council members certainly felt that this lack of individual preparation time before the meeting was a disadvantage. "It would have been useful to have the issue at an earlier time so that we could formulate questions in advance of the Council meeting", commented one citizen, echoing many others. "Not fully understanding the question", said one of the Council, "we were unable to ask leading [sic] questions immediately".

Was there deliberation?

It is clear that a combination of factors, but principally difficulties around the wording of the question, meant that the members of the Council found it hard to work with the information provided in the first meeting in the witness-based sessions. This section explores the review and small group sessions in more detail. These are the sessions where focused discussion, debate and deliberation might be expected to take place. It looked as though the design of the meeting allowed a reasonable amount of time for this. How were those spaces used in practice?

First, what, in practical terms, is meant by 'deliberation'? Chapter Two laid out the kinds of activities theorists include within this complex concept. In principle, deliberation can be a private cognitive activity, a calm musing and reflecting on facets of a problem to reach a wise conclusion. As a public collective activity, however, and in the sense used in Chapter Two, deliberation also involves collaborative work that may be anything but calm and quiet. Such work includes exchanges between two or more speakers around a common topic with back and forth reactions to each other's views; puzzling over an issue to work something out collectively; the sharing of reactions, for example, to witness positions; trying to understand the position of other members of the Citizens Council; and willingness to be persuaded by another's position. There is the possibility of disagreement, conflict and argument, and discussion of that disagreement. Ideally, all this discussion should lead to a possibly, but not necessarily, consensual resolution of or conclusion to the question being explored.

A qualitative account is necessary to capture the subtleties of deliberation in practice but a simple, pragmatic, quantitative indicator of the amount of deliberative discussion in this meeting was also developed, not least because it was then possible to compare across meetings to see whether changes in design made a difference. A minimal baseline definition of deliberation was devised. The number of standardised lines of transcript where there was an exchange between two or more speakers around a common topic and responding to each other's views was counted for all the review and the small group sessions (the only sessions where extended discussion of the topic was possible). It is a minimal definition in the sense that *any* exchange was included, even when not relevant to the question of clinical need. The percentage of the whole taken up by this form of interaction was calculated. As a reliability check, a second researcher coded a random sample to check the application of the definition. A perfect match was found between the coding of the two researchers.

Extract 3 below provides an example of deliberation taken from a small group session on the second day of the meeting where the members of the Council worked on a case study. This long exchange meets the definition used: it is a back–and–forth exchange around a common topic. It also includes the other features of deliberation noted above. Members of the Council are puzzling over the dilemmas presented by a case study and are trying to reach some kind of collective view on just what the priorities for treatment should be. Although the extract is quite hard to follow, it can be seen that they are listening and responding to each other's points and are beginning to discuss the reasons for disagreements so they can reach some kind of resolution.

Extract 3

Bridget: "I think for me personally, the reason is that the painkillers don't work, and they're in agony. So to me everything and they've got short, shortened lives so they should have a little bit of quality of life before they die."

Claire: "Mmm."

Bridget: "To me personally, you know.... I used to visit this little boy who had cancer. Oh and he was in agony. It was like a particularly painful form of cancer. He died. He was five when he died. And it was horrific to go there, and you'd hear him screaming with the pain. And they couldn't do nothing about it and that was awful. And I wouldn't like to think, you know, that anybody, if I never met them, was in that much pain that they couldn't have some sort of relief you know."

Teresa: "I think it's quite personal. Well, you can make it a personal thing because if you were.... Say your mother had, er, needed a hip replacement...."

Bridget: "Yeah."

Teresa: "You would want her to be given priority, but it ... looking at it dispassionately, if there was a child suffering from a form of cancer that needed huge amounts of money spending on it. You know you would, you would want that doing? But when you're looking, personally involved...."

Bridget: "Yeah."

Unknown: "It's difficult."

Unknown: "Yeah it's difficult."

Female: "Whatever it is that you're involved in, as far as you're concerned is the priority."

Bill: "Yeah."

Bridget: "Yes."

Teresa: "That's just human nature."

Bridget: "Yeah."

Teresa: "Yeah."

Bridget: "Yeah, they're difficult choices innit, they are. Because out of those choices we were choosing between them. The one that would get a news in the newspapers and would be popular would be the hip replacement. Because nobody would bother about the [unclear]...."

Very little of the interaction of this first Council meeting, however, could be described as deliberative in form, even by this most minimal of measures. In all, deliberation accounted for only 10% of the total interactions in the review and small group sessions. Why was the figure for this kind of back and forth around a common topic so low? Part of the answer undoubtedly lay in the problems the Council members experienced working with and weighing up the information given. "We are ignorant by design," acknowledged one citizen later, at the induction for new members after the third meeting; "we are there to ask questions". But "knowing what you think is damned hard; you'll change your mind every session!". This was not the whole story. The difficulty of the question set was certainly a factor. It is also important to note that the majority of the deliberation took place in the small group sessions. The size of the whole Council (*n*=30) made facilitation of deliberation very difficult in the plenary sessions.

Where does facilitation figure in this? In general, the facilitators of the Citizens Council chose an inclusive style of facilitation, making sure that all who wanted to speak could speak, usually in order of request. If we look in more detail at the content of the review sessions, we can see what this looked like in practice, and why as a consequence there was little deliberation in the plenary sites.

The facilitators typically organised the review sessions in the first Council meeting, and also in many of the small group sessions, around a flip chart. They encouraged members of the Council to summarise points from witness presentations and put them up on the chart – a practice favoured by moderators of citizens' juries in the US (Stewart et al, 1994). In the US citizens' juries, each juror is then asked in turn to explain his or her position on a particular point. The first meeting of the Citizens Council, however, did not follow this route (although the practice was adopted for some sessions in later meetings). Members of the Council were free to contribute points or to remain silent. And they contributed in the order in which their upturned name cards were seen by the facilitator.

Extract 4 below is taken from one of the review sessions. It illustrates the flavour of the proceedings, and shows why the organisation of these sessions might have stifled deliberation and debate. The extract comes from a session at the end of the first day.

Extract 4

Nigel: "He said learning. Learning to recognise the whole problem not just the immediate one, ie treating the patient as a whole, not just a condition. So when you mentioned about cutting out a brain tumour, but it was the after-effects and treating the whole person's depression, personality, everything."

Facilitator: "Okay, any other points that people thought were particularly key?"

Mary: "I ..."

Facilitator: "... from that?"

Mary: "Sorry, it was also one of value-based medicine rather than evidence-based. And not just jumping to a scientific thing. And while one set of criteria may indicate you have an illness another set might not, or something like that."

Facilitator [spoken to flip chart scribe]: "Are you keeping up, Shirley, or are we shouting these out too fast? Good on yer [background laughter]. Yeah, that's great. Emma and then Trudy."

Emma: "I don't know if I missed it when I was writing, if anybody said it, but he talked about making the best use of scientific evidence. Has somebody said that [muttering from background]?"

Woman: "Emma. But he did, he did say it."

Man: "Yes, he did yeah."

Facilitator: "Trudy?"

Trudy: "The diversity of human values."

Facilitator: "Yeah [background laugh] any other points from Professor [name]."

Faced with an uncertain task, which often came at the end of a long and demanding day, the facilitators and the members of the Council quickly settled into a reassuring routine for conducting review sessions. The emphasis was placed on *remembering* and *reviewing* rather than *discussing* the evidence. As Extract 4 demonstrates, this often involved attempts to reproduce the discourse of the experts and to utilise their terminology. Members of the Council thus suggested a series of points or statements they had picked up from listening to the witnesses that were either recalled or noted down at the time. These were then recorded on a flip chart. By the end of the session, many had contributed and quite large numbers of points had been listed, using many pages of the chart. Little else in the way of digesting or discussing had happened. Fragments of expert discourse remained as just that. The next chapter will return to this point: when does knowledge become a useful tool for a deliberative community of practice and when does it remain a foreign and unassimilated discursive 'Trojan Horse'?

This mode of organising review sessions encouraged an educative frame and a 'student' positioning of the Council. At times something akin to a 'quiz show' standpoint developed. The values guiding the contributions from the members of the Council became accuracy, memory and comprehensiveness. The task became one of trying to remember everything that had been said and little distinction tended to be made between points that had a bearing on the clinical need question, and arguments and claims about health issues and the NHS in general. The emotional tone of these sessions was good-humoured and relaxed but, as they continued, the observers noted that many of the members of the Council appeared to become bored and disengaged.

Deliberation would have been an altogether more difficult task, with the threat of disagreement and conflict, but it might have been more stimulating and more to the point. Interestingly, although some citizens were initially worried about conflict, several wanted to deliberate. "It would be nice to have more group debate", opined one Council member rather wistfully after the event. Another wanted "more time to allow the Council to discuss evidence as a Council with an open-floor general discussion and debate". From a facilitation point of view, however, chairing such discussion with 30 active participants is extremely testing. It was not surprising in the circumstances that the facilitators focused mainly on the rights of individual members to be included and to speak when they wanted.

Developing recommendations for the report

If this was the tenor of the interim review sessions, what would the final report be based on? "The only difficulty I see is getting thirty people to decide what we all agree on – that's going to be difficult", predicted one of the citizens in the round of interviews before the first meeting. A more serious danger, however, was that the report might consist simply of those points from the witnesses recalled by members of the Council. If so, NICE would merely obtain a somewhat imperfect record of the material that had been put into the meeting. Did a report emerge which presented an informed public's view? Since this is such an important question, the organisation of the final sessions will now be examined in detail. We will also trace the trajectory of one of the key recommendations in the report, that concerning age. It was the mention of age in the report from the first meeting that led to it becoming the topic for the second and third Citizens Council meetings. How did this recommendation first emerge, and what led to its inclusion in the report?

Perhaps unsurprisingly in view of what had gone before, the final sessions proved to be immensely difficult. The facilitators had considerable experience with citizens' juries, and the two lead members of the facilitation team were very skilled. As already noted, it is a challenging task to moderate a citizens' jury of 12 members discussing a clear yes/no dilemma, even when all participating thoroughly understand the issues. It is another thing to moderate deliberation on a poorly understood and complex topic with a Council of 30. As observers, the research team and the NICE project manager began to become aware that a lot of creative work would be needed to work out a design and format for future meetings of the Citizens Council so that it could meet its objectives.

Three hours on the last day of the meeting were devoted to developing recommendations on what NICE should take into account in its decisions on clinical need. First, members of the Council worked in four small groups, each aiming to produce three lists on flip charts: (i) on the features of the disease or conditions that seemed most important to them; (ii) on the features of patients; and (iii) a priority list of different stakeholders, picking up the sub-aspects of the clinical need question. The intention was that the lists on the charts should be consensual (or indicate points of uncertainty) and should sum up discussion in the small group. After the small group work, the whole Council would meet together to reconcile the separate lists and reach some final conclusions. Parts of this design worked smoothly, for example, aspects of the small group work, but the bringing together of the material from the groups in a plenary was not successful.

The final review session started with a member of each group reporting back on decisions. The facilitator posted up each group's flip chart on the wall and suggested that, as the delegated small group member read out each point, the Council should decide which issues they agreed on, and which needed further discussion. A tick was to be placed on the chart next to issues where there was consensus, a question mark where there was doubt and a cross if it was to be excluded.

The facilitator worked hard to maintain sufficient order. Part-way through the session, the Council decided it made sense to report and discuss decisions from each small group, question by question, rather than reviewing responses from one small group on all the questions. It was also agreed that, when a new small group presented their decisions, they would only report additions to the list. In practice, however, the revised procedure was difficult to choreograph. Feedback from the small groups tended to include everything on their flip chart, which replicated ideas and extended the process. The overlaps caused confusion for the member of the facilitation team charged with compiling a list agreed by the whole Council. Further confusion occurred when the delegated small group member quickly listed their group's decisions leaving no time for the Council to decide whether to assign that particular point a tick, question mark or a cross.

The intention was that the second half of the final review session would offer the opportunity to debate the issues that had been given a question mark. Items that had been allocated a tick were to be incorporated into the report. However, time became limited, so the facilitator suggested that the Council restrict itself to about two minutes for discussing each of the remaining topics. As a consequence, he was frequently forced to close down the debate. Extract 5 is taken from the second section of the review session and illustrates this process. It is clear that, due to this time pressure, there was little opportunity for weighing up evidence for the points where there was no consensus. Arguably these would have been areas of contention of particular interest to NICE.

Extract 5

Bridget: "It's not a clever comment. It's just that the question is, 'the important features of diseases or conditions' and genetical factors are important, aren't they?"

Facilitator: "Alan, then David."

Alan: "Exactly the same."

Facilitator: "Thank you. David?"

David: "Well I'm possibly the reverse. Does it matter whether it's genetic or anything else? It'll get looked at in the same way?"

Woman: "Yeah."

David: "The cause of it is irrelevant, whether it's genetic or otherwise."

Facilitator: "Rachel, then Nigel."

Rachel: "We're not talking about the cause of it. We're talking about, erm, if it's affected somebody in that family. Then everybody else in the family might need to be tested for it."

Man: "Yeah."

Facilitator: "Nigel?"

Nigel: "True, we're talking about what is clinical need, and whether it's genetic or not. It's nothing to do with clinical need. It's an illness; it needs treating."

Facilitator: "Two more speakers, and then I'm going take a vote."

Evelyn: "I agree."

Facilitator: "Sorry, no, two more speakers and then I'm going to take a vote on it. And I've got Jim and then Evelyn."

Although this review session was not the only source used in producing the final report, it was clear that it was going to give the facilitators a difficult task in producing a coherent, representative account of the thinking of the members of the Council. Not only was the design for the session not working, there was no pool of deliberative discussion to draw on from other sessions in the meeting. The problems can be seen clearly if the trajectory of the specific recommendation on age in the report is tracked.

The first mention of age in the final review session came when the second small group reported back to the whole Council. Extract 6 below shows how Guy, the member of the group delegated to report back, indicated that there was some debate over whether age might be important in discussing features of a disease or condition. The facilitator, who had also been the facilitator for that small group, then asks whether it should get a question mark. The response of the small group is confused, but one or two voices agree, and one member raises a question about whether Guy has accurately recorded this point. Discussion moves on to another topic at this point.

> **Extract 6**
> Guy: "One for the debate we had was age."
>
> Facilitator: "Did we, I think?"
>
> Bridget: [unclear]
>
> Facilitator: "Yeah, so shall we put a question two next to it?"
>
> New speaker: "Yeah."
>
> Bridget: "Yeah."
>
> Anoop: "Guy, have they got outcome on that sheet because I didn't think [yeah] I mean I can't tell because it...."

The next mention of the topic occurred when the Council moved on to discuss the sub-question about the most important features of patients in assessing clinical need. The first group to report back on this question seemed to be saying that their view was that age should be taken into consideration. In Extract 7 below, the transcript of this episode starts with the end of a decision-making process on 'hope'. Then Bill, as spokesperson for one small group, suggests that 'age' should be taken into consideration but swiftly moves on to mention 'social background'. This extract illustrates the confused nature of this session and how disorganised the assignment of ticks, crosses and question marks had become.

Extract 7

Facilitator: "It's either a cross, a tick or a question, Guy."

New speaker: "Cross."

Facilitator: "Is it a ... ?"

Man: "Cross."

Facilitator: "Bear in mind we've 15 minutes before coffee."

New speaker: "Yeah, cross."

New speaker: "Cross."

New speaker: "Cross."

New speaker: "Question, Guy."

Facilitator: "Question, Guy?"

Man: "See who can shout the loudest."

Man: "No one can shout louder than me! [laugh]"

New speaker: [unclear]

Bill: "Age should be taken into consideration, social background, state of mind."

Man: "Age, yeah."

Man: "Eh!"

Woman: "What's, what's social, I'm sorry, what's social background?"

> Woman: "I don't understand that one."
>
> Facilitator: "Somebody from that group want to unpack it a bit from [facilitator's] group?"

The brief discussion that followed summed up what the small group discussion had been about (a discussion of social background and means testing), and the point was allocated a question mark.

On both occasions in which age came up in the final session, there was major confusion over process and over the final view reached. First, it was flagged as a matter for further discussion with no consideration of how it might be relevant to assessing the important features of conditions or diseases. For the second mention of age, there seemed to be some consensus among the small group proposing it, but there was no discussion among the Council as a whole about this recommendation. In the second part of the review session, the issue of age was not discussed further. In the report, age was not mentioned under the section on features of diseases and conditions that was one of the two areas where it had been discussed in the review session. However, age was mentioned under features of the patient. The report included the sentence: "The Citizens Council felt that the age of a patient should be taken into account when deciding clinical need". Not surprisingly, NICE struggled with this enigmatic statement, and wanted further clarification on the issue.

The facilitators worked hard to ensure that the report reflected proceedings. They had to hand not only the flip charts but also the detailed notes taken by the team at the sessions. They sent drafts of the report to the Council members for approval at an early stage after the meeting. Taking the nature of these final review sessions alongside the material earlier in the chapter, however, it is clear that there must be major questions about the value of the report from this first Citizens Council meeting. Although NICE wished to use it as an indication of an informed public view on clinical need, it is not possible to conclude that it was a record of decisions reached after a visibly satisfactory deliberative process among participants in a position to thoroughly explore the issues.

Inclusiveness, voice and influence

Developing informed views and collective dialogue are key aims for a deliberative standing council. But even if the NICE Citizens

Council had been able to work well in these domains at its first meeting, the value of their efforts would depend on achieving a further very important goal. Hearing a diversity of voices and hence social inclusion is an important background ideal for deliberative democracy. The notion of communicative rationality, for example, developed by Habermas, constructs an ideal speech situation where there is no deception, domination or coercion of others. Even if this ideal is unattainable in practice, a forum should be designed so that all can contribute as equally as possible, and one where there is a quest to hear minority viewpoints. NICE took this requirement very seriously. From the beginning, social inclusion was prioritised as a key requirement for the Citizens Council, and Chapter Three described how the recruitment process was designed to produce an appropriately diverse Citizens Council. But what happened during the meeting? Did the proceedings allow all members of the Council to have an equal voice and influence? Were minority voices heard?

Several quantitative measures were developed to answer this. One simple and basic way of assessing level of participation was to measure the space each individual member of the Council took up in relation to the total contributions from all members of the Council. The number of standardised lines of transcript resulting each time an individual member spoke was entered into a database. Taking individual differences first, some quite marked variations were observed. Three speakers, for example, accounted for 25% of the total while at the lower end of participation it took around 14 speakers to contribute an equivalent 25%.

The size of individual contributions is not necessarily straightforwardly correlated with level of influence on the proceedings. Someone who speaks a great deal might not actually be 'heard' by the rest of the Council. Such individual differences in themselves are perhaps not concerning but a problem certainly arises if there are systematic imbalances related to the demographic characteristics of the Council since we can infer that the entire range of views might not be available to the group as a whole. Were there such differences? It is hard to draw firm conclusions from one meeting but we can take a first look at gender, at minority ethnic groups and at visual impairment.

In Figure 4.2 the percentages are broken down across the six main plenary sessions of the Council. It is clear that at the beginning of the first Citizens Council meeting, male members of the Council spoke more frequently than their female counterparts. However,

Figure 4.2: Participation levels of Citizens Council members by gender for meeting one (Clinical Need)

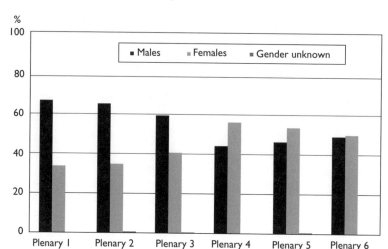

interestingly, this pattern changed in the middle of the meeting, with women contributing at a higher level than men in the second half.

There were two members of the Council with significant visual impairments. One of these members contributed at an above average level and one at a below average level. The contributions of the four black and minority ethnic members of the Council, however, were all below the average level of participation. The significance of this is difficult to judge for just one meeting and the next chapter will return to this question when there are more data to report. Similarly, although quantitative measures of inclusion play a useful role, they do not have the potential to answer the questions raised in Chapter Two about the domination of proceedings by hegemonic discursive styles. This issue and qualitative analysis relevant to its investigation will be a central theme in Chapter Six.

Importantly, the citizens themselves were for the most part satisfied at this stage that the facilitators had done their best to include everybody. Good practice included careful chairing of the meetings to regulate the amount of time taken up by any one individual, small group work to facilitate quieter members, tracking individual contributions during the meeting to identify those who had not spoken, and encouraging them to do so, and, later on, for the second Council meeting, one-to-one work with those struggling to find a voice to help them become more involved. Other forms of informal support that developed included helping individuals who were having difficulty understanding documents (relating to the witnesses) that were sent out in advance of subsequent meetings. Braille versions of most of the materials for Council discussions were prepared. Staff from Vision 21 followed up members of the Council who failed to show at any of the meetings and this often involved lengthy telephone conversations and support to catch up on missed meetings. On the face of it, then, and at this first meeting, the findings on inclusion look rather better than those relating to information and deliberation.

Conclusion

A successful Citizens Council, as with any deliberative forum, depends on orchestrating a range of variables and bringing them together in a 'good enough' manner on the day. The first meeting was derailed by several contingencies, including the wording of the question put to the Council and the design of the review sessions. The question certainly picked up a central (and familiar) topic for NICE, but it left the citizens 'bemused'. "It was rather daunting", said one of them later, "to be given a question to answer that NICE couldn't even do – especially at such short notice". Crucially, too, the design of the review sessions seemed to freeze out deliberation, arguably to preserve social inclusion. The casualty was a proper process for reaching recommendations for the report. But these matters of local design tap into much broader questions about how citizens are positioned in these kinds of initiatives, how organisations frame such events, the nature of deliberation itself and the foundations of the current enthusiasm for deliberative democracy which will be explored further in following chapters, and in Part III.

Meanwhile, for NICE and Vision 21, there were some immediate, practical lessons. It was a case of going back to the drawing board, redesigning and experimenting with the structure and organisation of the event over subsequent meetings. As one of the citizens concluded: "I suppose as it was a 'first', there are always areas that can be improved". And another reflected sanguinely: "I feel that we will be able to start from a better position next time we meet with the confidence gained from our first Council deliberations". The next chapter picks up these questions of design, examining the fruits of rethinking by the organisers and facilitators on the practices that should guide the Council.

FIVE

Better by design? Subsequent Citizens Councils

Despite the impression sometimes given of the 'naturalness' and spontaneous ease of democratic deliberation, artful performances are demanded from citizens, organisers and facilitators alike, if deliberation is to occur, and if its results are to be documented and put to use. Aspects of the design of the Citizens Council meetings changed following the first event, and there were further changes as experience began to accumulate. With different kinds of sessions, a different balance between them and different styles of facilitation in place, the focus of the analysis in this chapter is on the impact of changing design. Using the findings from the ethnographic investigation, we continue to explore the concrete case of the NICE Citizens Council to discover more about the micro-level conditions that impede and facilitate deliberative performances, building up a picture of the kind of community of practice that emerges and the nature of deliberation as a discursive practice.

Data were collected from a further three meetings of the Citizens Council – at Cardiff in May 2003, Sheffield in November 2003 and Brighton in May 2004. By the fourth meeting in Brighton, the Council had been 'refreshed'. Ten existing members, chosen by drawing lots, had left the Council to be replaced by 10 new members selected following the same recruitment principles. By this means NICE hoped to avoid members of the Council becoming institutionalised, their ordinary commonsense perspectives diluted as they learnt more about health debates. Quantitative outcomes were measured for the second and third meetings in Cardiff and Sheffield using the transcripts of the video records to add to the results from the first meeting. The records from the fourth meeting were included in the qualitative analysis, but time constraints prevented a full quantitative analysis. The research team was requested to give substantial interim feedback to NICE between the second and third Council meetings and this was a further influence on meeting design.

The first section of this chapter reviews the main alterations in the meeting format made by NICE and the facilitators. The second section reports some encouraging results from the quantitative outcome measures for the second and third meetings. The third section asks just why it was some of the changes seemed to work. It indicates how a finer-grained analysis of practice, resting on textual examination of transcribed speech, might both deepen understanding of the practices which go to make up deliberation, and begin to challenge aspects of the model of ideal deliberation. Rather than try to force practice into idealised theory, we need to develop theory to accommodate a growing understanding of practice.

Questions of design

The basic citizens' jury format chosen for the first Citizens Council meeting remained in place over the next three meetings. Members of the Council still worked on a question set by NICE; they listened to and questioned witnesses; they continued to work in small groups and to develop recommendations for a final report in a plenary review session. Nevertheless there was a lot of scope within this template for creative and constructive modifications.

Questions to the Council

Following up the enigmatic reference in the Citizens Council's first report on clinical need, the NICE steering group decided that the second and third Citizens Council meetings would both take up the topic of age. They introduced a two-meeting model, where both meetings would work on the dilemmas around age and the allocation of healthcare resources. The Cardiff meeting would reach some preliminary conclusions that could be revisited in Sheffield. For the fourth meeting the topic then changed completely: not only a new subject, but also a different kind of question. The wording of the questions put to the four Citizens Council meetings can be found in Box 5.1.

Box 5.1: Questions for Citizens Council meetings one to four

Meeting one (clinical need), November 2002
What should NICE take into account when making decisions about clinical need?

There are three key elements that NICE would like the Citizens Council to consider specifically. These are:

1. The most important features of diseases, or conditions, that should be taken into account when deciding clinical need.
2. The most important features of patients, rather than their conditions, that should be taken into account.
3. The weight the Institute should give to the views of each of the various groups of stakeholders (consultees) in deciding clinical needs.

Meeting two (age), May 2003

Are there circumstances in which the age of a person should be taken into account when NICE is making a decision about how treatments should be used in the NHS?

Supplementary questions:

4. If there are, what are the circumstances?
5. If you think there are circumstances where age should be a factor, in what ways should it be taken into account?
6. Should NICE value a year of an individual's life differently depending on their age?
7. Are there differences in the ways in which the cost-effectiveness of a therapy should be taken into account when deciding what treatment should be used for different age groups?

Meeting three (age), November 2003

Should we be more generous in our definition of what constitutes value for money for some groups rather than others? And, if so, why?

Should NICE be more generous in deciding what is value for money in these circumstances:

8. Where some age groups are at a greater risk than others?
9. If the treatment offers greater clinical effectiveness for some age groups?
10. Because people tend to have different social roles at different ages?
11. Based on how much people have time to experience life due to their age?

Meeting four (confidential enquiries), May 2004

Should the national confidential enquiries be required to seek prior consent from every patient and next of kin whose identifiable data are used in their research?

In answering this question the Council will need to consider, among others, the following questions:

12. Are the enquiries making an important contribution to health?
13. Is gaining patient/next of kin consent impractical and (for next of kin) too intrusive, or not?
14. Are the enquiries' current arrangements for ensuring patient confidentiality adequate?
15. Is the balance between the desire to gain consent offset by the benefits to the public of the enquiries, or not?

As can be seen, the questions became more concrete as time progressed and increasingly more embedded in the briefing papers that members now received, particularly so for the last meeting. This process was slow, however. Observation suggests that the questions on age for the second and third meetings were still too complex and abstract for participants, and members of the Council continued to express a lot of confusion and dissatisfaction at those meetings (although it had markedly reduced by the third meeting). In terms of format and formulation, the most successful question was the one prepared for the fourth meeting.

Without a doubt the significant factor here was the actual discursive construction of the question and the kind of answer requested. As one citizen put it, looking back at the topic of age:

> "The question as drafted was poor. Instead of such a direct question, an open style would have relaxed the concern over ageism. For instance, start it: 'NICE would like to hear the Citizens Council views on…'."

Crucially, to whom was the question addressed? What kind of 'audience' or respondent did the question construct? Was the ideal respondent a moral philosopher, for example, or a final year medical student? As Box 5.1 illustrates, the questions seemed to presuppose and address an 'every person' expert audience, where the task was to find a universal answer or set of moral perspectives. By the third and fourth meetings, it became clearer that the Council's task was to work out their own view (as a notional 'public') where there might be other competing views, and not act as some kind of an omniscient ethical adjudicator on all relevant perspectives.

Similarly, the questions varied in the range of the dilemma posed. The first Council meeting had started very broadly indeed with clinical need, which arguably related to virtually every social value consideration relevant to NICE. The second and third meetings then narrowed this down to one specific aspect. The dilemma was still phrased, however, in complex terms such as 'year of an individual's life', 'value for money' and 'clinical effectiveness', where a good answer would depend on a sound understanding of those complex technical terms as mediators of the basic ethical dilemma. The questions for the first and second meetings asked for recommendations on circumstances, factors and features. They assumed a fine-grain response was possible, with qualifications, distinctions and precise specifications for different aspects of the dilemma and for different contexts. By the fourth meeting all of this had dropped away, leaving a much more narrow and direct formulation of the ethical scenario. The questions were being put in a yes/no format which seemed to be much more productive: should something be done or not? It seems likely that as a result a much more successful 'expertise space' had been constructed for the Council. A space might be emerging, in other words, where the Council could be empowered and competent, which might make the best use of their time and knowledge base, and which took a realistic view of the amount of complex new information and qualifying aspects which could be covered in a three-day meeting. Chapter Six will come back to this important issue of how citizens become disempowered when 'expertise spaces' are misjudged.

Commensurate with this new approach, NICE modified its own relations with the Council. For the first meeting, NICE took a 'hands off' approach, not wishing to bias members. In line with natural science thinking and the gold standard of randomised double-blind trials in medical circles, the steering group's concern was about avoiding 'contaminating' the results of their experiment. But, to be effective and properly independent the public needs to understand just how they are placed, in this case as an advisory group to NICE. Ignorance of their real position (they were not there as the recruitment advertisement had suggested to 'have their say' about the NHS) had impeded their work. In the third meeting particularly, NICE took a much more extensive part in the proceedings, explaining their own activities and giving much more background to their interest in the question. By the fourth Citizens Council meeting, after this experience, an extensive induction for the 10 new recruits, and a different kind of question, NICE could again drop into the background, with the Council much clearer on their role and their function.

Witnesses

Given participants' impressions of the directionless flavour of the witness sessions in the first meeting, and the low levels of focused questions, some redesign was necessary. For the second and third meetings the number of external witnesses decreased markedly. Nine witnesses gave individual presentations at the first meeting in Salford and there was one NICE panel presentation with three speakers. In Cardiff there were six individual presentations and one three-person NICE panel. By Sheffield there were only five external speakers and two of these were from NICE. The overall space given to external voices and to the process of informing the Council remained fairly constant across the Council meetings as a proportion of total activity, but the nature and role of the witnesses changed.

One innovation in the second meeting, for example, was to introduce witnesses who were very clearly positioned, for or against, on the age dilemma. An excellent example of this was when the Council heard from a health economist and then a gerontologist with totally opposing views. The health economist presented an argument for intergenerational inequity, or what he termed the 'fair innings' view. He argued that the young should be favoured where there were scarce resources, since older people had already had their 'fair innings'. In contrast to this, the gerontologist presented an argument for equity and for judging people on their abilities and their physiology, rather than on the basis of age. In the third meeting, further innovations to the witness sessions included a video presentation from the National Children's Bureau (NCB) so that the Council could take account of the voices of children and young people. Witnesses also started to become more creative in their presentations. Another health economist, responding to the situation, for example, developed a very effective back-and-forth interactive session with the Council to replace his planned lecture.

Interestingly, the fourth Council meeting returned to the traditional format of relatively large numbers of witnesses. It was felt that because the question was so specific, it was important to make sure that the members of the Council were properly briefed on the background to the issue. There were six external witness presentations and three panel presentations. Unfortunately, the balance of information was open to challenge. Four of the witnesses came from the national confidential enquiries, arguing, unsurprisingly, for exemption of these enquiries from the need to gain informed consent. Those who took an opposing stand included a solicitor with a background in a voluntary organisation for victims of medical accidents, and a junior barrister. Effective presentation of this latter position was arguably made particularly difficult given the continued presence of the confidential enquiries witnesses throughout the meeting. Some of them had told the Council that if they were to be forced to gain consent the enquiries might be closed down and they would lose their jobs. Council members were alarmed by the responsibility. Their feedback forms also showed that they were aware of an imbalance of views. "We could have done with a bit more of the 'anti-attitude' to the big question", one person wrote. Another form included the comment "there should have been 50 per cent for and 50 per cent against".

Small group and review sessions

Several innovations were introduced in the small group sessions, particularly from the third Council meeting onwards. The size and patterning of the groups became much more varied. Members of the Council, for example, were asked to work in combinations of twos and threes around the main table, as well as in the more usual three groups of 10 in separate breakout rooms. Activities with twos and threes included working on a particular part of the question, reviewing previous sessions and coming to some conclusions about how they would answer the question prior to the final review session. A further change in small group work in the fourth Council meeting offered members the opportunity to nominate their own issues for discussion. Those members who nominated a topic sat in various parts of the plenary room, while the other Council members freely moved from group to group discussing the chosen issue. Increasingly, the trend was not to facilitate smaller groups. The hope was that without a facilitator there might be more space for the members of the Council to debate and argue.

Work with case studies was greatly increased in later Councils, and was often combined with role-play. For example, in the second meeting the members of the Council were split into four groups and asked to play the role of one of four sub-committees of a local health authority board. They were told that the health authority had been given an 'Aid Innovations' grant to spend on new treatments, and had to decide which treatment to favour. Each group was asked to make a case for a different treatment and, after they had presented these cases to the Council as a whole, the floor was opened for general discussion and a collective decision on how to spend the money. This pattern of intensive small group work followed by a structured debate was replicated in the fourth meeting, while the third meeting included a mock NICE appraisal committee exercise. One effect of these modifications was to blur the distinctions between witness presentations and small group work. Formats were pragmatically mixed as necessary.

In the later meetings, the membership of the facilitation team was adjusted to place more stress on deliberative facilitation, particularly in the review sessions. A new facilitator was introduced in the third Council meeting, who acted not only as an additional 'living dictionary', but also led sessions challenging the Council to identify and focus on key issues and differences of opinion, pulling these out wherever possible. His role was defined as that of 'devil's advocate': he was there to ask witnesses the questions that the Council members had not known to ask.

Plenary sessions became much more diverse and stimulating, with further new and creative tasks added around the edges. For example, a new activity called the 'lucky dip' was introduced at the beginning of the third meeting, with the aim of easing the members of the Council back into the mindset of ethical debate. One of the facilitators moved around the plenary room inviting members of the Council to choose a moral dilemma out of a hat. The person first read out the dilemma, and then had to say what they would do in that situation, with the Council as a whole then discussing it.

A further activity in the same meeting involved an array of photographs representing diverse individuals of varying ages placed around the walls of the coffee area. Members of the Council were handed 'play money' at several points over the course of the meeting that they could allocate (through placing the money in boxes under each of the photographs) to the individuals whom they thought worthy. The aim was to demonstrate that people change their minds over the course of the meeting as a normal part of the deliberative process. In the fourth meeting, the facilitators introduced questionnaires based on the question posed to the Council for members to complete at various points over the course of the meeting. Again, the idea was to demonstrate that council members changed their views on the topic, and these changes were reported back to them. This meeting also introduced the notion of a 'reflection period', where members were given a space to think through the issues for themselves.

Significantly, the process of arriving at recommendations also became much more transparent and organised. Before the final review session in the second meeting, for example, members of the Council were asked to work in twos, and write down their thoughts on the question together with their reasoning. They then worked in small groups to prepare recommendations for the final review session. The format for making recommendations was thus centred less around voting and ticks and crosses against witness points on a flip chart. It gave more emphasis to drawing out the reasons behind the members' decisions, even though statements of these reasons needed to be fairly brief. The process of producing the recommendations in the final session of this meeting was still fairly chaotic, however. It was still a very difficult exercise to facilitate such a large group so they could reach consensual decisions, or even clarity on disagreement.

In the third and fourth Council meetings the final review sessions began to place much more emphasis on each individual's response to the question, with a greater focus also on individual writing tasks. In the third meeting, for example, members were asked to write their responses to the question individually, and to provide qualifications for their decisions. These responses were then posted up on the walls around the meeting room for everyone to read. In the fourth meeting, members of the Council were again asked to write down their individual response to the question, and then asked to discuss their reasons in small groups. The small groups then reported back their recommendations in a final plenary session. These individual writing tasks enabled facilitators to incorporate individual views into the report in a much more systematic fashion. Contributing to, and ownership of, the report were very important for Council members. The production of their report on the topic was the reason they were there:

> "I always feel proud after we've actually ... finished the report, 'cos I'm like ... I've done something – and it's been worthwhile."

> "You feel like you've achieved something. I think we all do."

Overall, however, the notion of deliberation guiding the design of the Council was shifting from a predominately collective to a more dispersed act; this included individual and paired ruminations as the organisers dealt with the implications of facilitating a large group of 30 through to some consensual conclusions. The report would now serve more as a record of opinions and preferences after collective discussion than as the coordinated statement of a public arrived at through whole group dialogue that rehearsed contrasting points of view and resolved differences.

Outcome measures

What was the impact of these changes in design? In the previous chapter, two simple quantitative outcome measures for charting patterns in the interactions of the Citizens Council were introduced: the number of focused questions, and the percentage of lines of transcripts in the small group and review sessions which met the basic condition for deliberation (back-and-forth exchanges on a common topic, not necessarily relevant to the question set). Levels of participation were also measured to assess social inclusion. What did these measures reveal now?

Focused questions

The percentage of focused questions increased markedly across the three meetings – from 28% in the first meeting to 57% in the second meeting and 56% in the third. In effect, the proportion had almost doubled. This was a much more reassuring picture for NICE and Vision 21. It demonstrated that interventions in the design of deliberative assemblies can make a difference, and suggested that the various modifications, particularly in experimenting with the number and style of witness presentations and the format of the question, were on the right lines. This improvement in the number of focused questions was also appreciated by the citizens, some of whom had privately expressed frustration at what they had seen as 'irrelevant' questions put by their peers.

But despite the increase, these figures suggest that the Council was still struggling to work with the information presented. A large proportion of the questions to witnesses remained unfocused and irrelevant to either the witness presentation or the core question being discussed. Does this matter? Some communication researchers (for example, Hewes, 1996) have suggested that group discussions are inevitably and naturally incoherent and it is unreasonable to expect anything else. Hewes argues that group members do not in general strive for coherent discussion because they are more concerned with formulating their own thoughts about the group decision, rather than responding in a relevant way to what has gone before. A group member's utterances, in his view, are "thoughts out loud" with the more solipsistic goal of helping the speaker think through the issues. Speakers are thus merely thinking in the company of others rather than truly adding to a cumulative body of thought.

From this viewpoint, the NICE Citizens Council is simply doing what every group does. This argument, however, has been discredited by other communication researchers. Pavitt and Johnson (1999), for example, closely followed the discourse of 62 small groups, examining relevance criteria not dissimilar to those used in our measure of focused questions. They found that there was strong evidence that groups were indeed communicating and were engaged in coherent discussion. Although different measures were used in the Pavitt and Johnson study, the number of groups was fairly large and the data suggested that a group typically does show more coherence than is evident here, rendering the large percentage of unfocused questions in the Council a matter for genuine concern.

To describe a question as unfocused does not mean either that it was unimportant or that the members of the Council were in some sense deficient. The issue is how the deliberative space was framed and constructed and whether this was done in such a way that the Council could actually engage and fulfil their brief. The large percentage of unfocused questions for the second and third meetings was probably due to continuing problems with the formulation of the question put to the Council. Although without the ambiguities and difficulties of defining clinical need, the questions for the second and third meetings were still quite convoluted. Had the questions on age been formulated in the crisp and clear yes/no fashion of the question for the fourth meeting, it is likely that the proportion of focused questions would have been even greater. Unfortunately it was not possible to compute a quantitative measure, but qualitative observations from the fourth meeting suggest that there was a further marked increase in focused questions as the format of the question crystallised. The next section will explore in more detail why changes to the witness sessions also seem to have made a difference to this aspect of the Council's practice and gives hints about what might have been possible if the question had been better formulated.

Back-and-forth exchanges

Just as the number of focused questions doubled, so too did the amount of back-and-forth exchanges on a common topic. This mode of interaction, which is a basic condition for public deliberation, constituted just 10% of the small groups and review sessions in the first meeting. In the second meeting it increased to 21% and to 25% in the third meeting. This again strongly suggests that the modifications introduced by NICE and Vision 21 were working. The trend was upwards, with a clear increase between the second and third meetings. Qualitative observations of the third meeting indicate that the increase was more significant than the figure of 25% suggests. The third meeting achieved a very different deliberative mood from earlier meetings, while the fourth meeting improved again. Measurements of the back-and-forth exchanges in the review and small group sessions, although still important, became less useful and reliable as time went on and the different kinds of activity of the Council began to blur into one another. More interactive witness sessions meant, for instance, that these too sometimes became occasions for dialogue. And the third meeting included periods where members of the Council, working in twos and threes, discussed the issues among themselves and it was not practical to record all of these for later quantitative analysis.

How should the quantitative pattern for dialogue and discussion be evaluated? Despite the positive trend, and the possibility of under-reporting, the percentages still seem low, especially given the minimal nature of the definition of deliberation used. Should not a lot more space in a Citizens Council be taken up with back-and-forth exchanges at those points where this kind of dialogue is possible? Would one not want to see a higher proportion even if the goal of the Council was simply to encourage individual thought and reflection on the issue to reach an informed opinion? Caution is needed in interpreting these findings. There are no comparative norms. What would count as an appropriate percentage, let alone an ideal figure? Perhaps a figure of around 50% might indicate a healthy deliberative forum? Obviously, a great deal depends on the quality of the exchanges. Even a figure of 10% might be satisfactory if the exchanges were highly focused, generating high-quality debate at just the right point in the proceedings, and producing an agreed set of recommendations or a novel clarification of different positions for a report. In practice, however, some of the dialogue that met the 'back-and-forth' criteria was not about the set topic at all, but about other matters, such as how the policy for 'retirement' of councillors should be handled. Furthermore, the discrepancy between the qualitative observer reports for the third meeting and the percentages for that meeting suggests that a numerical figure can only be a rough guide to the health of the proceedings. It establishes whether the necessary condition for a deliberative assembly has been met, but can tell little about the productiveness of those exchanges in relation to the topic. The next section will utilise more qualitative analysis.

Levels of participation

Turning to social inclusion, as in the first meeting, there were substantial individual differences in levels of participation. Throughout all three meetings, a small group of councillors contributed at a much higher level than others. Over time, members tended to fall into relatively distinct groups, as high contributors, average contributors or (a much larger tail of) quieter contributors. Whereas the high contributors tended to remain relatively consistent in their level of participation across the first three meetings, the quieter contributors were more· variable. Marked differences in individual levels of participation are to some extent inevitable but might be considered a problem if quieter voices are being silenced. Ethnographic observations suggest that usually this was not the case. Most people who wished to speak managed to do so, frequently at the point in the meeting where they wanted to do so.

Members of the Council did from time to time express some dissatisfaction or a feeling that a few people were overly dominant, and that "some find it harder to get their voices heard":

> "There was a few times that [the facilitators] did allow it to get, not out of hand, but sidetracked, and people talking over people, and she wasn't following the proper [procedure, where if] you've got your [microphone] light on ... no one else talks. I won't say [that she] lost control but it became hard work to get your point across because people were speaking to each other over the tables ... and that got annoying because then you see the quieter person slowly withdraw again, just as you felt they were coming out of their shell."

But mostly those with the highest levels of contribution tended to be highly valued, and their contributions were positively received.

Little resentment was evident and little notice taken of their greater level of participation. The previous chapter noted that Vision 21 developed strategies for supporting individual members of the Council who might have had trouble contributing. Certainly, some members expressed their appreciation of the ways in which 'turn-taking' was facilitated in the plenary sessions, which enabled quieter people to overcome 'the hurdle' of speaking in public:

> "We have our name card, because then we can turn [it] rather than everybody fighting [to speak] on top [of each other] ... which is good. The first meeting for me ... as I don't have experience in a big meeting like this ... [was] quite daunting. But I've passed that now ... [and if] I've got a question, a point to put forward, I can raise my hand – which is nice."

Only one member dropped out of the Citizens Council altogether. His participation rate was initially low and declined, although it is not clear whether this was the cause of his withdrawal.

There were some interesting differences in participation levels in the plenary sessions compared to the small groups. Contribution to the plenary sessions was more asymmetric than the contribution levels in the small groups. In other words, in the plenary sessions a smaller number of people spoke rather a lot, with a longer tail of members of the Council who spoke less. The distribution for the small groups was flatter and more symmetric. Small group work is often recommended as a way of increasing the range of contributions to public debate in comparison to more formal plenary sessions. This seems to be borne out for the NICE Citizens Council. But, turning now to the patterns for gender, ethnicity and for some of the members with disabilities, it will become clear that not all voices were equally enabled by small group work.

Gender differences were relatively small in scale across the three meetings. The pattern evident for the first meeting continued in subsequent meetings. Male members of the Council tended to take up more space than female members but not greatly so, and female members of the Council tended to contribute more in small group than in plenary sessions. Male and female members participated on relatively equal terms, however, and the differences were not large enough to suggest a systematic or extensive pattern of exclusion based on gender.

What was the overall experience of the two members of the Council who were visually impaired? When data were combined for all three meetings, it was clear that as in the first meeting the members of the Council with visual impairments were able to contribute in the plenary sessions at levels comparable to other members, and better than average in one case. This was not true, however, for small group work. The contributions of both members with visual impairments dropped markedly from plenary sessions to small group sessions, and their average contribution in the small group sessions was less than for other members. For members of the Council with visual impairments it was a significant disadvantage to be placed in small groups.

Why was this? It would appear to be connected with the fact that these small groups were often not facilitated, or facilitated in a very variable and not very effective way. Indeed, several Council members themselves commented that these groups needed to be "supervised" or "chaired" by active facilitators. "They are too open to being dominated by one particular viewpoint; I found that I had to back off", said one member. Small group work tended to be much less disciplined, and the resulting melee of voices made it very difficult for visually impaired members to find the right moments to gain the floor. In addition, briefing materials needed to be translated into Braille, and this was patchy as overheads and PowerPoint produced on the day were often not translated. For very obvious reasons the use of the flip chart as the main focus for small group work and the device of 'post-it' messages also significantly disadvantaged members with visual impairments.

Finally, the participation levels for the four black and minority ethnic (BME) members of the Council were compared with the average participation level for the Council as a whole. The contributions of the BME members were muted and significantly lower overall. These results are worrying but difficult to interpret. The sample is small, and the patterns could be due simply to individual differences. It could also indicate, however, systematic bias and lack of success in creating a situation where BME members felt their contributions were welcome. There were very few BME expert witnesses, which may have had some effect on this outcome. Qualitative observations suggested that either (or a combination) of these interpretations might apply. There were certainly some significant problems within the Council in this area and the following chapter will return to this issue and discuss in more detail the dilemmas the Council faced around inclusiveness.

What makes a difference?

The quantitative measures have suggested that, although there were mixed results and many remaining issues, attention to design can make a substantial difference to the practice of a Citizens Council. By the end of the third meeting, the data suggest that the Citizens Council was working more effectively as a deliberative forum than was initially the case. The idea was that members of the public would consider complex issues of social value at the core of the Institute's activities, weigh up relevant evidence, viewpoints and information, discuss the issues among themselves, and reach informed and reasoned conclusions based on collective dialogue and deliberation. The factors that prevented this happening were clear from the last chapter; most obviously they were lack of clarity around the topic, along with review sessions that closed down dialogue and discussion. This section will look more closely at the factors that empowered the citizens in subsequent meetings – the patterns underlying the improvements in the quantitative picture reported above.

Interactive and positioned experts

Consider, first, the following extract.

Extract 8
Facilitator: "Thanks very much. Margo and then Harvey please."

Margo: "There are two things I want to say. First of all, well, I think you are wrong. My mother has just had her 70th birthday and last November she remarried and her husband is 80. He has cancer and we obviously would like to see John get all the treatment he can have to prolong his life as long as possible. They are out on holiday at the moment and for me this is the first time in 30 years that my mother has of having any happiness at all. So to us and to her it is extremely important that, you know, John is kept healthy and kept alive as long as possible so that they can enjoy what time they have left. So I think you are wrong in that respect. Old people do have a right to as much life as possible, we should try and treat them."

Health economist: "Ah yes, but as you see, as the quotation said, it is always a misfortune if you want to go on living to be cut back. But the question is suppose it was you or your mother? So we put it as a question of equity between the generations. What do you think your mother would say if it were you or your mother?"

Margo: "Yes, that's, I don't think age comes into that then does it?"

Health economist: "Well, it does between the generations."

Margo: "Yes, I mean if my mother was 20 and, you know, I had just been born she would feel like that but ..."

Health economist: "No, but you see I think you see I am not, as I have said several times. There are lots of very beneficial things you can do for old people, no question about it. And presumably the treatment your mother is having at the moment is successful, it is working and it is cost-effective. Okay, that is fine. But the question is, suppose the resources have got to be shared? Somebody earlier asked a question about these three pills, you know. I mean that is the extreme, that is the extreme case kind of thing, would you not be influenced by the interest of intergenerational equity what point in somebody's life they are at."

Margo: "[Exasperated sound] I hear what you are saying and maybe it is from a selfish point of view as well, but from my own personal point of view I would like to see John's life prolonged for my mother because ultimately when John dies my mother then becomes our responsibility as a family [laughter]. Yes, it is from a selfish point of view. But the knock-on effect of what happens, you know, it really sort of snowballs over quite a few families."

Health economist: "But as your previous witness said at the very end ..."

Extract 8 comes from a session in the second meeting questioning a witness. Margo is not asking a question, she is engaged in what could be described as a deliberative back-and-forth exchange with the witness, using a personal story to challenge his point of view, and arguing with him. Unlike the question to witness sessions in the first meeting, this piece of interaction is highly engaged, is on topic, and both participants are actively digesting and reflecting on each other's arguments and viewpoints. As noted in the first section of the chapter, one useful innovation in the second and third meetings of the Council was to introduce witnesses who were very clearly positioned, for or against, on the age dilemma. The health economist above was a witness of this kind, developing a 'fair innings' case for diverting resources away from older people. As we have noted, he was paired with a gerontologist who argued against any form of age discrimination. Margo, in the extract above, is challenging the notion of 'fair innings'.

Interestingly, the sessions where witnesses presented a strong for-or-against position also tended to produce the highest number of focused questions. A highly positioned argument tends to be easier to assimilate. The points made refer to each other, and the sequence builds to an obvious conclusion. Crucially, a clear and highly positioned witness presentation allows the audience to engage with the views expressed and stimulates them to work out their own response. There is a much higher level of attention and investment.

Equally, witnesses adopting an interactive style were usually very effective in encouraging the members of the Council to work with the information presented. Sessions which modelled and displayed the different possible positions which could be taken on the question seemed much more useful than sessions which summarised the evidence per se. One example can be seen in Extract 9 below; it comes from a witness session in the third meeting. Although it is part of a longer exchange, we can see the general style adopted. Instead of giving a formal presentation, the witness covered a number of issues in an informal dialogue with the members of the Council, handing the floor back to them after he had raised, and briefly discussed, each issue. He was also very clear in this session about his own personal views. Here, Hilary, in a back-and-forth exchange with the witness, gets him to clarify his position. The level of emotional and intellectual engagement with the witness and his position is very different from the 'set piece' questions more characteristic of the first meeting. (Note that in this extract the numbers referred to are years of life.)

Extract 9

Teresa: "Well I was just going to say something that Harry's just said, which was that the 70-year-olds have actually been 20 and been 40. I take it a step further and say the 40-year-olds have been 20, the 20-year-old has only had 20 years of life so far. Having said that my first reaction is to say it shouldn't be on age at all. But that would, if faced with that (and that was the only choice you had) that would be my decision?"

Facilitator: "Okay I've got Hilary, Joan, Guy, Anoop, er Susan?"

Hilary: "I think you should have had 60 rather than 70 up there 'cos it makes that even more emotive I think. And you say you wouldn't choose the 40 if they were single. But supposing they were the only person in the family who was earning and had dependent parents or disabled siblings or something, then what will you do?"

Facilitator: "Okay."

Hilary: "Over to you?"

Health economist: "Oh, you want me to answer? Well is it? See it.... This is where I've tried to make these questions macro-group level questions rather than individual bedside questions because ... and I've got sucked into individual bedside by you. Because at the individual bedside there probably are many things that we might like to find out when faced with very difficult organ transplantation. But I may wish to take account at the individual bedside, but I might not want NICE to have a general principle on. And I think that's the difference. So I've been ... let's find out all we can about them when it's an individual clinical, an individual bedside decision, where I can see the whites of these three patients' eyes. But when it's a macro-level group level decision I would feel very uneasy about a general principle...."

Hilary: "Well, that's precisely why we shouldn't make a distinction about ages then. You just said that."

Health economist: "No, no, no, no, no. Because at a general macro-resource allocation decision level I'm entirely comfortable with NICE saying ..."

Hilary: "Everybody over 40 shouldn't get ...?"

Health economist: "Not at all, not at all. I'm entirely comfor—"

Hilary: "You just said that."

Health economist: "No, no, no, no, no, no. Let, what I haven't said, I haven't said that at all. I'm entirely comfortable with saying that in the absence of other information. I wish and it's a stated policy goal within the NHS. Since you're asking my own personal view that we should, wherever possible, do the most with the limited resources we have. And 'do the most' in this question, will mean giving 60 years of benefit for someone as opposed to 10 years of benefit to someone else. Now if the ages were the other way around I'd still make that judgement. I mean you'd be living to 130 if you were 70 and you'd be living to 30 if you were 20. I'm not using age in that example, I'm not using age as my criteria, I'm using the expected benefits from treatment."

What this extract suggests is that, although there are still issues to consider about how the introduction of experts positions citizens and frames democratic deliberation (cf Wynne, 2005), and Chapter Six will return to these, in later meetings of the NICE Citizens Council the professional discourses of the experts began to be meshed dialogically with the life world discourses of the citizens. In the first meeting, expert information was treated more deferentially and gingerly. It was not successfully assimilated into the emerging discourse of the Council. As the previous chapter demonstrated, it was simply 'reviewed', remembered as isolated points and facts to be put up on flip charts rather than worked over as living arguments.

The fate of the 'fair innings' case is testimony to this point. It became a standard reference point for the meeting; it was frequently cited and seemed highly influential. But, fascinatingly, the members chose not to support this argument in their final report. "He gave an extreme side of the picture," explained one member afterwards; "having been privileged all his life, I felt he didn't put the views of someone who had done hard physical work all his life and who wanted to enjoy a long and exciting retirement and deserved the opportunity". The collective assimilation, assessment and rejection of the 'fair innings' case is positive evidence that, provided with the right materials, a Council can work with complex information, challenge it from their own points of view, and make recommendations. It is also reassuring for the status of the final report. If the members were presented with a clearly articulated argument that they engaged with and then rejected, there can be more confidence that the report reflects the view of a diverse group of informed citizens. Whether it would be representative of citizens as a whole, a debate taken up vociferously within NICE as Chapter Seven will show, is a different matter.

Emotional investment

One of the distinctive aspects of the NICE Citizens Council is that the brief was to reach conclusions about general (and rather abstract) social values. Members of the Council were selected because they had no particular personal stake or vested interest in the likely issues under discussion. In contrast, as Chapter Three noted, most citizens' juries work on highly specific policy issues (for example, where should a new motorway be sited?) and members of the jury are sometimes drawn from the constituencies with a strong stake in the outcome (Pickard, 1998). Several authors now argue, contrary to the image of rational, calm and 'sanitised' deliberation, that emotional investment in the issue oils the wheels of deliberation. With such investment comes the motivation to discuss, and to engage with, material and with fellow citizens (Lowndes et al, 2001; Barnes, 2004).

Our findings support this claim. The NICE Citizens Council, as the examples from Margo and Hilary above demonstrate, engaged in more focused discussion and in exchanges which were more deliberative in style when the content under discussion concerned concrete cases and when they were responding to strong invested statements from witnesses and could identify and mobilise their own strongly held opinions in response. One of the reasons why experts with a clear position created more coherence and focus is that they brought about strong emotional responses in their audience. They polarised and clarified an otherwise rather vague and confused ethical picture.

As Chapter Two noted, many of the early advocates of deliberation were inspired by a contrast between the kind of environment found in 'politics as usual', and the environment which might be possible in democratic deliberation. 'Politics as usual' was oppositional, antagonistic, highly rhetorical and emotionally manipulative. Democratic deliberation could be more reflective, more rational, less egocentric and more focused on collective good. This image also guided the planning for the NICE Citizens Council and the aim of providing a reflective space which would bring out the best in citizens, where they could have an opportunity to work out what they might think when they had as much information as the experts.

As experiences have accumulated, however, advocates of democratic deliberation have become more pragmatic (for example, Johnson, 1998; Dryzek, 2000) and much less prescriptive about ideal modes of communication. Critics, too, such as Iris Young (2000), have convincingly argued for the appropriateness of emotional displays and the inclusion of more diverse modes of discourse. Our findings support this trend. On virtually every occasion, as the topic got more concrete, relevant and focused on an actual real-life issue, deliberation in terms of our simple quantitative measure increased.

Deliberation also increased whenever citizens themselves were assigned a position to argue, and when they could emotionally identify and invest in the outcome of a discussion. The abstract discussion of ethical dilemmas was much less compelling. It was still the case in the second and third meetings that more often than not questions to witnesses and review sessions failed to lead to extended dialogue, but there were at least some tantalising hints of styles and strategies that might provoke more engagement.

Deliberative facilitation

What else might help a group of citizens 'weigh up' and deliberate? Further clues are contained in the extracts above. A common focus sustained over several turns in a conversation is crucial. This is easiest in a dialogue between two people, as Extracts 8 and 9 demonstrate. When large numbers of people become involved in the conversation, and the floor passes from speaker to speaker in relatively rapid succession, there is the danger that the topic will shift or become diffused. It is also crucial that there is permission for people to engage in an extended back-and-forth discussion while others listen. One of the advantages of the session in Extract 9 was that the witness gave Council members that permission.

A key issue here is about how best to facilitate. The tension between inclusive and deliberative styles of facilitation that surfaced in the first meeting continued to be an issue in subsequent Council meetings. With inclusive styles of facilitation the chair's task is to make sure that everyone gets a chance to speak, and that the scarce resource of addressing the Council is rationed evenly between the members. Other tacit 'rules' operate: for example, that each member can only ask one question and that the ideal at the end of the session is for all the councillors' questions to have been asked rather than a few explored in depth.

Extract 10 below demonstrates how members of the Council began to organise their conduct around these implicit rules. The extract comes from the second meeting: the question session with the gerontologist witness mentioned above, where he argued against any form of age discrimination. In this extract, a member of the Council asks a question, and a contentious point is raised by the witness in response that probably needs further discussion. Instead of responding to the reply from the witness, however, the member of the Council continued with another question. The members of the Council had learnt that one way round the 'rule' was to ask a question with several parts as that gave them more time to interact with the witness. While interaction was sustained, the discussion of ageism had been terminated. Other members of the Council did not have the opportunity to pick up this topic or any other aspect of this particular answer from the witness either.

Extract 10

Facilitator: "Thanks very much. Fred and then Bridget."

Fred: "I have enjoyed your comments. Two questions. The first one, what words would you put in place of ageism, what words would you put, in well, the terminology in place of ageism?"

Gerontologist: "I don't want to replace the word yet. I think it is a deeply useful reminder that there is an underlying social prejudice that feeds into all this thinking about it. I mean the classic example I am always being asked oh there is one lifebelt and two women have fallen into the pond and one is aged 18 and one is aged 80 which one do you give the lifebelt to? The fact that everybody thinks that the question can be answered in any other way than if one woman was black and one woman was white is a clear indication that people don't realise that ageism is as deeply rooted as racism was 20 or 30 years ago. So it is a useful concept. I will be glad to see when it becomes obsolete."

Fred: "Right, the other part of the question is this...."

Is this a real problem? One could argue that the function of the witness session is to impart information. If that information is discussed in a later review session, for example, or reflected on in private, then perhaps it does not matter that there is little public and collective weighing up of the information among the Council during the question sessions. This conclusion is not persuasive. What happens to the information in these cases? It is as though the arguments presented by witnesses, and emerging in their answers to questions, become suspended. The information is left hanging, waiting to be used at a later point. It may never reappear, and people forget the points they wished to make and their reactions at the time.

A better solution might be to combine inclusive and deliberative styles of facilitation for all sessions, and to set the explicit and implicit ground rules accordingly with the members of the Council. The members of the Council need to be given permission to ask a question, then to respond to the reply, and for that avenue to be exhausted before moving on to the next question. This, of course, is a much more demanding kind of facilitation. Equal opportunities need to be maintained and close attention paid to the conversation to judge when the dialogue is productive, when it is complete, and when another question is needed. The advantage is that the imparting and the weighing up of arguments and information can occur in the same session.

Arguably, a more deliberative facilitation style can be seen in the next extract, certainly in the sense of encouraging a run of thought to develop. In the third Council meeting, the sessions that produced the largest amounts of back-and-forth exchanges occurred when members of the Council worked with two members of NICE in mock appraisal committees. These sessions were role-plays and were an exercise rather than the actual deliberation the Council would need to conduct on the age questions. The deliberative style generated was not translated into the business proper, but these sessions provided useful practice and some indication of what it takes to produce a back-and-forth dialogue with a large group around the same topic.

The chair of the NICE appraisals committee prepared the citizens by first giving a very clear presentation on what the appraisal committee was trying to do, and how it worked. He then offered a guide to a particular treatment that they were to discuss in small groups as a mock appraisal committee. The focus on Cox II inhibitors for reducing pain in arthritis for those in different age groups made the task 'real life', immediate, important and concrete. The citizens divided into two groups, one of which was run by the chair while the programme director facilitated the other. Extract 11 shows the latter guiding the members of the Council in a discussion about the suitability of the treatment for different age groups. Together the group jointly worked towards some recommendations.

Extract 11

Programme director: "Now got this dilemma about this issue."

Bill: "We should guideline to slow down."

Programme director: "Is there any ..."

Bill: "Not to use the Cox II."

Harvey: "'Cos we know that they're not suitable for anyone."

Bill: "That's right."

Harvey: "I mean they appear to be. We came in here. I'm sure people approach.... I heard saying 'Oh this is the answer, yes. I can have those doctor'. Now we know a bit more, a bit more information."

Programme director: "They're not, they're not necessarily suitable..."

Harvey: "No."

Programme director: "... for everyone. It looks like there's some evidence about the types of people that they're suitable for. But they've not quite enough evidence in other circumstances. So where does that leave you with thinking about what sort of recommendation you would make of it?"

Nick: "There isn't much choice. Recommend, you say, in general with reservation. And then it comes down to the, well, giving it. Provided your doctor has sufficient information in order for him to decide whether in fact he does prescribe them."

Programme director: "Let's talk about those reservations then. There's a proposal, 'use in general for some people'. That's going to be a good idea but ...."

Nick: "Yes."

Programme director: "What are those things. So let's have an exploration of what the 'but' might be?"

Graham: "Well from a cost-effective point of view we're already told to treat all patients works out at hundred and fifty thousand per life year gained."

Programme director: "Yes indeed."

Graham: "So you're in effect ... as NICE you'd be looking to slow that down anyway."

Programme director: "So, on a cost-effectiveness basis it doesn't look like it's cost-effective just to recommend these for everybody?"

Margo: "Not for general use, no."

Programme director: "And ..."

Margo: "So it has to be for people who have a previous history of problems with ulcers or whatever who are not at risk of ..."

Graham: "Cardiovas—"

Margo: "Cardio problems."

What the programme director is doing here is holding the frame and topic for the group, bringing the discussion back to key points and unresolved issues, using questions to the group to do so. Accounts of reasoning thus surface. The dilemma (which will be discussed further in the next chapter) is that this type of facilitation can become a guided discussion set by the facilitator's agenda, and there is a risk that a particular hegemonic professional discursive style comes to dominate Council members' styles. Typically, the facilitators for the NICE Citizens Council did not attempt to control the topic in this way. By allowing people to speak in strict rotation with little intervention, the topic would wander from speaker to speaker and there was no sustained focus. Extracts in the previous chapter demonstrated what this looked like in practice and why it did not produce deliberation. This then is another nettle to be grasped. Not only is it the case that people might deliberate better when emotionally engaged, but also they might become more empowered when facilitators are more active in managing the topic – but with the danger of loss of alternative modes of reasoning and alternative understandings of the topic.

Conclusion

This chapter has documented a range of changes that were made to the initial design for the Citizens Council of NICE after the experience of the first meeting. It has demonstrated the impact of redesign by comparing the baseline measures of witness questioning and deliberation that were taken for the first meeting with those achieved subsequently and it has concentrated on transcripts to tease out what makes a difference. The citizens themselves, interviewed after meeting four, were, for the most part, satisfied that the Citizens Council was now a success. It seemed to them that their feedback had been heard, ways of working were improving, and they themselves were "getting better at the job":

> "The last meeting was the best; it went very smoothly. The rapport between us all; we're not wasting time any more, and there's not the babble of wasted talk.... We're very much getting down to the information at hand. So ... the whole thing ... has changed and we're a lot more effective I think."

The measures that we had devised lent support to this – in the sense that there were now more focused questions and more indications of the back and forth of deliberation than in the first meeting. Changes to the design indicated that this was more than a result simply of growing familiarity and confidence. More specific and concrete questions and more imaginative techniques for information sharing and digesting, for example, are recommendations that recur in the commentaries on and assessments of juries. The design changes had moved the Citizens Council rather more in the direction of a citizens' jury, although the initial conception of the Council as needing to be 'at one remove' from the daily business still limited the extent of travel along this path.

With an opportunity repeatedly to revisit and reflect on the transcripts, what more has emerged? And what does it say in relation to the successful conduct of deliberation? There were certainly moments in the four meetings that operated like a deliberation theory textbook. Citizens were engaged, passionate, arguing well, with consideration for each other's viewpoints, focused on the big picture as well as the details, exercising their collective voice, noting the disagreements and highly motivated to see beyond their own preferences to some more inclusive standpoint. We linked these with strongly positioned witnesses, meshing dialogically with citizens; we showed the power of emotional investment and opened up the question of different modes of facilitation. But moments of deliberation were rare. They happened in fragments and at unpredictable times – in witness sessions for example, rather than in the review sessions designed to open up a specific deliberative space. They also happened most often to one side of the main business – in role-plays, for example, and when citizens were debating questions of procedure (such as the retirement policy for Council members themselves) with their hosts. For all these reasons, the case for developing a 'bottom-up' understanding of the nature of deliberation as a social practice was becoming more compelling.

Chapter Six continues to analyse the material, providing a more sustained account of the councillors' discursive styles than hitherto. In doing so, it highlights issues of power, interests and identities that have concerned sceptics among the ranks of deliberation theorists.

Power, discursive styles and identities

The last two chapters tracked through the Citizens Council meetings chronologically, generating a blow-by-blow account of how one community of practice grappled with the challenge of democratic deliberation. It turned out to be a much more contingent process than anyone might have suspected (including perhaps a deliberation theorist). Deliberation emerges as fragile, as proceeding in fits and starts, as requiring a large amount of thoughtful nurturing and as permeated through and through with dilemmas of inclusion, control and engagement. This chapter, the last one using ethnographic data from the Council meetings, returns to some of the broader issues discussed in Chapter Two raised by critics of deliberation and the sceptics. These were concerns about power – both overt attempts by dominant groups to control the agenda and subtle effects of hegemonic discourse. There were also issues about interests and expertise, and there were questions of identity.

The first section of the chapter looks more closely at the terms through which the voices of minority ethnic group members of the Council were included in the Council and there are issues here about negotiating pluralism relevant to any deliberative assembly. The second section then examines some of the discursive styles deployed by members of the Council to deal with the new context they found themselves in, and picks up the question of the influence of hegemonic discursive genres. Finally, we turn to the nature of the 'citizen identity' in contexts where experts are present and citizens are 'being informed'. Can a collective citizen voice emerge within such a frame? Overall, we engage with some of the implicit and explicit social-psychological assumptions contained in the conventional models and ideals before outlining in Part III a new conceptualisation of deliberation as a dialogic discursive practice.

Pluralism, ground rules and 'politeness'

One key aim for deliberative initiatives is that they entail more than a conversation among the like-minded, simply validating participants' existing views. A deliberative forum tries to construct a group with diverse interests, positions and life experiences representative of the diversity of the wider population. Through engaging with different viewpoints, respectfully listening and being open to persuasion, a better and more inclusive solution to a dilemma might arise beyond 'business as usual', reflecting more than just the standpoint of any one interest group. As critics of deliberation have argued (see Chapter Two) this ideal of genuine engagement under conditions of equality is all very well in fantasy but perhaps unlikely to be realised in actuality. Are clear ground rules enough to secure this ambition? Can a principled process ever be robust enough to combat the power of dominant voices and interests? Here we offer a qualitative assessment of this issue, going behind the scenes, to add to the picture gained from the quantitative measures of levels of participation reported in previous chapters.

For BME members, the old, the young and the disabled, the NICE Citizens Council fitted a group structure which Kanter (1977, cited in Oetzel, 2001) has described as *skewed* (minority members are 1%-15%), rather than *tilted* (minority members are 16%-34%) or balanced (minority members are 35%-65%). The Citizens Council was a majority of minorities, so to speak, but with many key minority groups there in small numbers. Participating with 1%-15% of people who share core aspects of your social identity and social location, whether that is in terms of ethnicity, age, sexuality, disability or regional identification, is a very different experience, inevitably, than participating in a group which contains 65% of people who share your social identity.

It is not just a matter of whether one is included but also *the terms* of that inclusion. There were several incidents in the NICE Citizens Council meetings illustrative of the 'terms' emerging for minority groups in this forum. One such moment ('the clapping incident') came at the end of the first meeting in Salford. We include a full transcript in Extract 12 below for the insight it casts into the difficult issues that need to be negotiated around inclusion in deliberative assemblies. As Extract 12 demonstrates, the incident began with one of the visually impaired members (Mary) referring to a disagreement with another member (Rachel). Rachel then went on to outline her view at some length. Although her point is complicated by the details of the earlier discussion, Rachel's position seems to be that minority ethnic and disabled groups 'play the system', and any special treatment they receive in recognition of disadvantage is not fair. At this point a number of the members of the Council applauded her stance loudly. Although Mary, the member with visual impairments, had a chance to reiterate her actual argument, and despite the plea by Trudy (a member of the Council from a BME group) that the group discuss this issue through, it remained unresolved, and indeed there was no further time for discussion. This was an unhappy conclusion, and it left the minority ethnic and disabled members of the Council at odds with the majority. One can speculate that they might well have felt excluded from the group at this point.

Extract 12

Mary: "Actually there's another. Me and Rachel had an argument at the end and we came up with a thing to disability and stuff. And also I thought may be ethnicity and things. To take that kind of stuff into account, but not to do it just for the sake of doing it. But only where it's relevant and not to discriminate against people on grounds of it so which is quite complicated."

Facilitator: "Le-le-let's bring Rachel in and if we don't resolve it we'll put a question mark next to it, it's one of them that is with social issues, ain't it, I think."

Rachel: "The argument that me and Mary had was ... Mary actually sort of slightly made a joke slightly I don't, you know. She says that if, when it comes to doing things you would, if being blind worked in your advantage, then you would use it. And if it worked in your disadvantage then you wouldn't use it. And I took offence to that because being white, being healthy, being young, people like me – okay I am a woman – get put to the bottom of the pile. And I thought that it's not fair that, erm ... I don't mean any offence to anyone in the room or anything like that. It's not fair that people use ethnic minorities, disabilities when it suits them. Don't use it when it doesn't suit them [the majority of the group claps loudly]....."

Woman: "Okay, so shall we put a question mark next to it? And come back to it [laughter] after the ..."

Joan: "... cop out [group laugh]...."

New speaker: "Right [...] age?"

New speaker: "... we've got that in...."

Joan: "... we've got that ..."

Mary: "... and [group laugh] ..."

Mary: "Can I just say as well, the illustration Rachel and I had was that if we both broke our leg she wouldn't want me to get all the treatment just because I was blind for instance and her to get hardly anything. Because we'd kind of be equal. But if it were with a hearing thing I would genuinely have more need because of my visual impairment to get it sorted out. So I think it is a factor but you can't just use it 'willy-nilly', do you know what I mean?"

Mary: "I ...."

Rachel: "... but when it's relevant ..."

Mary: "... yeah...."

Rachel: "... but not just as a white wash ..."

Rachel: "No I agree. If it was something for your hearing, perfectly fine. If it was something that you know affected you more than me, fair enough. But just to get things to go in your ..."

Rachel: "... not, not just to get things done...."

Mary: "... advantage then...."

Facilitator: "... and similarly with their ethnicity...."

Facilitator: "Okay."

[...]

Facilitator: "Yeah and I want to make sure that everybody wants it in. But Trudy, then Nick, I think have indicated on that."

Trudy: "It's strictly me come back to a statement again. This is speaking as the individual because I'm part of the group and because I want to have my voice said on many different grounds. I'd like to think that the health service that I pay into is going to be sensitive to me according to all of my needs. And I think it's something that we kind of need to argue out as a group. I don't know if we just need to spend ten minutes and everybody chuck their thing into the arena or whatever but I think it's something that I'd like to. I don't know how everybody feels about it, it is some issues that have been brought up I feel very passionately about from the induction. And also from some statements that have been made over the past couple of days. But it's something that really needs to be hammered out, I think that's just me personally ..."

Facilitator: "Yeah. Fair enough Trudy. We're gonna just complete this. We're gonna do question 3 after Guy's done, question 3 should be easy. It's about listing the stakeholders and putting pharmaceuticals at the top of the list etc [laughter] (cheapskate). Only joking. But after, and then we're gonna have a comfort break and there is no tea and coffee with that comfort break I've been led astray, there is none, you won't get that till four fifteen."

As it happened, Trudy was unable to attend the next meeting of the Council. Further pondering of the issue occurred among the rest of the Council also, and one member had this to say about joining in the clapping when interviewed subsequently:

> "I applaud this [ie the initial statement] in company with most of the Council and would most certainly not have done so had I thought that her remarks were in any way discriminating. Was this the case of 28 members getting the wrong end of the stick or just the two?... Perhaps we need to discuss this problem at the next meeting."

In response to this incident, the facilitators spent time with Trudy, and the NICE project manager resolved to present a further session on 'ground rules' at the beginning of the second meeting. The Council were asked to discuss in small groups what they would do if they felt somebody was being racist, sexist, heterosexist or derogatory to people with disabilities, or discriminating on the basis of religion. The NICE project manager challenged the Council to think about how they could discuss issues of this kind without upsetting any other member of the group. This was a difficult session to conduct and, again, we reproduce in Extract 13 below quite a long segment of the resulting discussion, as it poses sharply the dilemmas involved.

Extract 13

Nick:"Well, in that case I'll [all talk at once]. Well, the first thing we wanted to know why have we been asked this question?"

Wendy: "What was your topic?"

Male: "Racism."

Female: "What's your ...? Were you racist?"

Female: "I think we're racist."

Nick: "Racism. Yeah. Why have we been asked this question? And we wondered whether in fact there had been any complaints so far by the members of the Council about the comments or remarks that may have been made, that might have been interpreted by some people as being racist? Are you going to answer that for me? [inaudible due to background noise] And the other point though is that we think we should make a choice, all of us, between extreme racism and on the other side of the extreme political correctness. In other words we should, we should endeavour to agree what is the middle road. And lastly, and probably most important of all, we actually deny we ever said anything about Wales [laughter]."

Female: "Oh. So, yeah, any comments [inaudible due to background noise] ..."

Graham:"I think I've already expressed my view to you. But I believe we've been spending time here discussing political correctness when we're here to discuss the NHS."

Project manager: "Yeah ..."

Graham: "And unless, you know, I haven't seen any yes it's sexist or whatever views but I do worry that I ... the first day on the Council my first thought was I really hope this ... we're not going to be bogged down with political correctness. And I just worry that we're spending time and effort on this and maybe I don't see the bigger picture but that...."

Project manager: "Well, I can tell you, and this is speaking from NICE's point of view, we don't want to see you bogged down in political correctness because this isn't about being politically correct. This is about being able to challenge each other, have discussions openly about various issues that are perhaps ... and various views that may be held quite strongly by individuals. But also that some individuals may be upset by, hurt by somebody else expressing the view. But to actually say, 'how do we deal with that?' because at the end of the day what we want to come out of that is something. And when we're talking about values you can't, you're talking about all these things that go to inform values so in a sense how can we deal with it in the best way that doesn't ascribe to issues round being absolutely politically correct. And as I described it to you it's about being 'oh this is too sensitive a subject so shall we just brush it under the carpet under the guise of political correctness' or the other extreme that some of you have already talked about. And if you are, you are right, it is about finding the middle road and finding the best way to actually deal with some of that."

Graham: "I just worry that sometimes. I mean we already dealt with this in a case study, in I can't remember [inaudible]. It must have been Manchester [inaudible]. The case study on kidney dialysis I think. And one of the clients was a black middle-aged lady. And normally such comments, strangely enough the only person who touched on it is here Trudy, isn't she ..."

Project manager: "She's not here Trudy ..."

Graham: "And basically we're going to, well the fact that she's black doesn't even come into it. So we're already dealing with those issues."

Bill: "Yeah, I think we, we're intelligent enough to decide for ourselves and we all live our lives in different parts of the country. We all mix with different people. I'm sure we're intelligent enough to decide for ourselves how to treat something like that."

Graham: "Yeah, but whether you could [all talk at once] for reference is that you're now for everything [inaudible] when we've kind of already dealt with it."

Project manager: "I'm not saying anything about political correctness. I'm just saying when there are issues that are uncomfortable. And distinctly some people feel uncomfortable, some people feel upset, how do you want to deal with them? There could be things that lie outside political correctness."

As Extract 13 demonstrates, several members of the Council reframed the discussion as 'political correctness', and several also clearly resented what they defined as being told what to do or how to behave. These various positions and responses threaded through the following meetings and were still salient to members of the Council when they were interviewed six months later. There were members who appreciated what was attempted: "It would be helpful to set up this exercise on a regular basis", wrote one later. Another person singled out this session as a good memory. And another pointed out that this type of session should have been done earlier: "Something like this should have been done after the Manchester [Salford] meeting" following up the initial work on ground rules done during the induction of the Council.

Others, however, were uncomfortable, asking what had provoked it and "what did we do wrong?". One woman said:

> "Everybody said that nothing had particularly instigated that, but I know that there was sort of like a feeling that perhaps something had been said at the end of the first meeting that may have triggered that. Now, if that was the case I felt that it was perhaps bringing it back up again, instead of letting sleeping dogs lie type of thing. So, that was one point that I thought perhaps, did we really need to do that? I wouldn't say it's a bad memory, I just feel that, it may have been done better, or whether it needed to be done at all."

Another person described herself as "quite disconsolate" over this as she went to her room that night:

> "I felt you know, why are we here? We don't seem to be giving NICE what they want. Are we here to give NICE what they want or are we here to give an honest opinion? I felt that the whole of that evening really didn't give a good lead. People felt they didn't want to do it, you know; I'm sure you've got the footage and you'll find that people didn't want to discuss what we were discussing, and they didn't really know why we were discussing it. It was only that evening; in the morning, everything seemed to sort of come together again, although I honestly feel that we never really got the nitty gritty that we got at the first meeting. It

came back again at the last one a bit, but not to the whole degree I felt."

Group cohesion seemed to be one concern for these members of the Council. And many assumed that cohesion and a positive group atmosphere depended on covering over disagreements ('letting sleeping dogs lie'). This conclusion was heightened by the concern that some issues and differences were too dangerous or threatening to discuss. The councillors also reported guilt at having done something wrong, combined with resentment that they had been taken to task (as they saw it) mixed with doubt about whether they really were guilty. In other words, issues about social justice and cultural respect had become transposed in the Citizens Council into matters of personal relations and individual blame. From this standpoint, good practice seemed to consist in not noticing or commenting on the fact that someone was black, for example, while attempts to name and address difference were undermined and ridiculed as 'political correctness'. Clearly, it is extremely difficult to raise these questions and not be heard as judgemental, and to raise them without provoking guilt, hostility and anxiety in those felt to be judged.

Not surprisingly, the discourse of the majority of the members of the Council around 'race' reflected wider themes in British public and political discourse (Reeves, 1983) and themes in western white majority cultures more broadly (Wetherell and Potter, 1992). Equality was defined as identical treatment, and the majority ethos was that everybody should be treated the same regardless of colour, for example. Everybody should be treated, too, as individuals on their own merits and, as a consequence, any 'positive discrimination' for a group was unfair. This perspective was very evident in the following comment on the retirement procedures suggested by NICE for the Council. This member of the Council was adamant that there was no justification for special measures to ensure representation of specific groups:

> "I was all for the 'names in a hat' system but then I heard it had been changed to reflect ethnic balance. Would one member have been removed if there were two people of the same ethnic source pulled from the hat? I doubt it. In my book, we are all British and that should be enough."

As BME groups have argued, inclusion dependent on the 'largesse of the tolerant' (Husband, 1986) places BME groups in a very difficult position. Own definitions of identity go unrecognised as they are subsumed into white British culture. The assumption that it is polite and considerate 'not to notice' that someone is black is highly offensive if it is assumed that being black is problematic in some way which should be 'politely and kindly' ignored. In addition, BME groups experience the difficulty of appearing to argue against strongly held egalitarian social values through asking for recognition of difference.

What can be learnt from these incidents? Here several different elements combine: concerns about group cohesion, fears over disagreement, worries that difference will spiral out of control, guilt, defensive resentment, a particular definition of equality and particular discourses around positive discrimination and 'political correctness'. This combination of elements is doubtless not uncommon and suggests that wider social inequalities are likely to be routinely imported into the very fabric of a deliberative forum. As Iris Young (2000) suspected (see Chapter Two), more often than not powerful groups are likely to dominate the definition of the common good. Domination is subtle, though, as the example of the NICE Citizens Council illustrates. It may be done more through notions of 'good manners', worries about the group getting along without conflict, and not understanding what is at stake for minority groups as a consequence of the discursive resources available to participants, rather than crude attempts to seize the agenda and repress other voices. The members of the NICE Citizens Council worked hard on a personal level to support each other and to make every member feel welcomed and included, but the majority also consistently resisted the notion that minority group members might need a space to articulate their difference. For many, 'British' was a good enough description of collective identity and collective interests.

Reviewing evidence from group communication research for its relevance to deliberation offers one approach (Mendelberg, 2002). In relation to the specific points at issue here, Oetzel (2001), for example, reports that increased cultural diversity in a group is good for group creativity (using measures of group performance in work situations). This research has also demonstrated, however, that compared to culturally homogeneous groups, culturally diverse groups experience higher amounts of what group communication researchers call 'process difficulty', meaning tension, competition, conflict, misunderstandings and so on (for example, Watson et al, 1993). While strategies such as regulated turns at speaking and positive chairing to facilitate all voices are a basic condition for handling such 'process difficulties', they are unlikely to be sufficient. Similarly, recruitment to ensure diversity and a representative Council, although crucial, is not enough for the proper representation of all views. A forum could still be described as dysfunctional if the representation of groups has been achieved but the full representation of views is inhibited. Inclusion, then, we can now see, has to be proactive. It is a matter of monitoring and challenging the majority ethos, as the NICE project manager attempted. Creative new ways of exploring and challenging dominant views need developing – such as working with the assumption that personal inclusion (liking and respecting people as individuals) represents enough social inclusion, or that assertions of difference are dangerous because they threaten group cohesion.

Those designing deliberative assemblies are presented with a difficult conundrum. As one of the councillors asked (see the quote above): "do NICE want the Council's honest opinion, or if they don't want that, what do they want?". NICE did indeed want the councillors' honest opinion but they also wanted to support members of the Council from minority groups. Majority rule, strictly interpreted, would seem to imply that any racist assessment (or 'honest opinion') expressed by the majority would have to stand as the Council's democratic conclusion. This conundrum is perhaps more apparent than real. In practice, democratic and non-democratic spaces intersect and depend on each other. Democracy depends on non-negotiable rules, social structures and social organisation. As one of the facilitation team commented in a joking aside during the Sheffield meeting: "I like democracy when I am in control of it". Some control is necessary for a useful event to occur, including when required 'politically correct' interventions, although there may need to be considerable clarity about where the negotiable democratic space (open to majority rule) starts and non-negotiable ground rules (preventing some modes of expression) end.

Power and discursive styles

The power dynamics of democratic deliberation affect not just the terms of inclusion for minority groups and minority points of view; they are also woven into mundane decisions about the very styles of discourse to use. This section considers this issue of discursive style or genre in relation to power, influence and authority.

As Chapter Two described, the academic and policy literatures set up some relatively elaborate prescriptions for deliberation. A number of eminent advocates and critics have told us what deliberation, public consultation and strong democracy *should* and *could* look like (for example, Habermas, 1984, 1987; Young, 1989,

1990, 2000). The ordinary public, however, who become members of a Citizens Council, have for the most part not read Jürgen Habermas or Iris Young. That is, the public do not know the theory, the rules and prescriptions for deliberation, except in the various forms in which concepts of democracy and schemas for public participation have trickled down into everyday ideologies and practices. As a consequence, for the members of the Citizens Council, the question of how to deliberate is pre-eminently a practical rather than a theoretical problem. Little was known in advance. What would be appropriate? How should a Citizens councillor behave?

In working out how to deliberate, members of the Council drew on habits of social interaction derived from their communities, workplaces and families, combined with models and patterns derived from other sources such as watching debates on television. Here we look at four such discursive styles before considering more systematically the relationship between style and influence.

One interesting discursive practice adopted by some councillors was to take up what could be called a 'researcher speech style'. It was a creative way of trying to minimise the uncertainty involved in discussing topics where one has no recognised expertise. This discursive practice consisted of bringing facts or 'did you know' pieces of information to the group. These pieces of information would draw on expertise outside the Council or some evidence that had been read or picked up elsewhere. One member of the Council made a habit, for example, of cutting out extracts about medical topics that seemed relevant from the newspapers in the months in between meetings, and bringing in a file of these to the meeting.

Extract 14 is an example from the second meeting in Cardiff, in a session in which members of the Council questioned the former chief executive of a patient support charity. Unfortunately, these 'did you knows' from members of the Council were often only tangentially useful as they were not responsive to the argumentative line developing right here in this context, and would lead the witness off on to further fact giving, often about areas not relevant to the question the Council was discussing. But this was one definition and way of deliberating, and at the root of it was a desire to bring something positive to the table.

> **Extract 14**
>
> Fred: "Alright [name]. I just want to ... I've got a report here it's been in the local papers. The main heading is 'single vaccine for brain diseases'. I dunno if you have seen this report. Basically what it is, is a single vaccine could soon prevent the development of incurable brain diseases including CJD, Alzheimer's Disease also it could forestall Alzheimer's, Parkinson's, CJD, Huntingdon's and type G diabetes. The comment was also given by [name] the research director of Alzheimer's Society."
>
> Witness: "Excellent man [laughter]."
>
> Fred: "And his comments were that he hoped that the jab would be tested on patients, and could be at work within the next 18 months. What are your comments on that?"
>
> Witness: "Well that piece of research is very, very interesting, Alzheimer's Disease is caused, well one of the causes ..."

A second discursive practice frequently adopted was of deliberation defined as 'a barney' or a passionate competitive argument. Here an everyday speech practice – the fight and verbal sparring – was brought into the public forum. When it occurred in small groups, it quickly became highly invested and bad tempered. One of the disadvantages of adversarial discursive practice is that it typically becomes an exchange between just two protagonists and other voices are drowned out. It is also a situation where only one speaker can win and the other becomes a loser, and so resolution is difficult. In the plenary sessions, there were some exchanges of this kind between members of the Council but the chairing rules prevented escalation beyond a couple of turns.

Members of the Council also developed for plenary sessions a more sanitised and less interpersonal version of 'the fight', often self-consciously or self-referentially modelled on adversarial television and parliamentary debate and hard-hitting interviews. Clichéd phrases like 'let me finish', or 'let me tell you where you are wrong', and robust humorous putdowns signalled this quoting. This was an example of the kind of ventriloquism discourse theorists such as Bakhtin (Morson and Emerson, 1990) see as a standard part of discursive life. We are always quoting in everyday talk. Sometimes such citing and borrowing of others' voices and words is clearly marked as reported speech ('he said, then she said', 'he went like …'), and sometimes the source disappears as the other's voice becomes absorbed into our own (Maybin, 2001).

Extract 15 below is a short example of this kind from a plenary session in the second meeting where small groups were defending their corner in a role-play. Alan's longer intervention used some of the classic devices of political oratory such as contrast structures, lists with the same beginnings, extreme case formulations, personal attacks on dissenters, and so on. In this extract he puts down a new speaker (who is indistinct and unidentifiable on the tape). The laughter of the Council is partly at Alan's audacious riposte. But, throughout this session, laughter also seemed to indicate the Council's pleasure at their skill in reproducing the genre of hard-nosed debate. Arguably, they were admiring a good piece of amateur dramatics.

Extract 15

Alan: "I think first of all your scare tactics on the SARS didn't work by scaring us all that we would all end up in bed. Neither did the blackmail tactics work in the SARS case…. [inaudible due to laughter] the osteoporosis is. For cold being a bloody nuisance, it is not a nuisance to the GP when his surgery's full of old people with colds. It is not a nuisance when their hospitals are full of old people with colds. We are proposing this prevention of this ever happening again, not for a year, 10 years, wipe it out completely. Once this injection has been given to the old people and following on, the old people you will never see them in a hospital with a cold again."

New speaker: "If I can just differentiate, can we just differentiate between the common cold and 'flu, hospital beds are not full of people with common colds they are full of people with 'flu."

Alan: "I am sorry I didn't know that was your medical training was." [laughter]

New speaker: "There is already a vaccination for 'flu."

Alan: "Expert witness there is a GP sat with us who says beds are taken up with complications resulting from common colds."

Facilitator: "Might not be the cold itself, it is things that come with it."

New speaker: [inaudible] [laughter]

The third example we picked out could be called a 'chair of the committee' speech style. This was a less frequent but nonetheless discernible and significant discursive practice that translated expertise in other areas of life into the Council meetings, and was only open as a result to a few members. Again, it appeared to be a transposition of a tried and tested way of communicating that worked effectively in other contexts to answer the new challenge of how to operate in a Citizens Council.

Extract 16 below exemplifies this practice. In this extract, which came at the end of the first meeting in Salford, the speaker has been asked to address the chief executive of NICE on behalf of the Council. The style he adopts, therefore, is very appropriate. The practice of speaking as the 'chair of the committee' sets up a powerful summarising position. It involves speaking on behalf of the group as a whole, defining the agenda and their views. Usually such a practice is both focused on the task, arguing for one position presented as 'what we think', and is about creating a positive socio-emotional tone through reference to this consensus. Disagreements, diversity of opinion and minority points of view can become homogenised with the risk that they will be written out of the record.

Extract 16

Facilitator: "Okay that's smashing. Right, [name], we've, erm, exhausted everyone I think but despite that I can't believe the energy that was in the room, in the last few hours. [laughter] I thought by keeping everyone tired and up late and doing all sorts of stuff it'd be fairly passive when we came to the decisions. But oh no, it's been some heated debate. So I think a couple of the Citizens councillors want to give you a flavour of the debate that we've had. Is that okay?"

NICE chief executive: "Sure, pleasure."

Harvey: "Okay [name]. What it is ... first of all, thanks for coming and seeing us again. What we're saying now is what we're saying in the press statement and nobody shot us down a few minutes ago, when Anoop and myself said it. First of all it's been absolutely fascinating. It's been a learning curve like you wouldn't believe. We've been totally entranced. We'd like you to arrange a half an hour's personal consultation for all of us with the clinical specialists we've met [laughter] 'cos we think we need it. We'd like to say some very good points. First of all the way that [chair of NICE] and [name of expert witness] walked in and said, 'right forget all this nonsense of these titles'. 'You know my name's so and so'. Wonderful start because it's not only crediting us with being human beings but also it's a way of communication and we very much appreciated it. Very, very impressed with nearly all of the speakers with a proviso that it would have been very nice to have some coalface people turn up. Wendy mentioned paramedics, you know absolutely, you know because I'm sure in answering some of the questions that are going to come up, it'd be nice to have these people here and a nurse. And it would not only help us. Sorry?"

Woman: "We had a nurse."

Harvey: "We, oh we had a nurse, but someone out of clinical practice."

Man: "Yeah not a working nurse."

Harvey: "She wasn't a working nurse. Everyone agrees. She wasn't a working nurse. So somebody that's actually handling patients and it would not only help us, it would actually give a bit of credit for NICE to be talking to people at the coalface, so we think that's good. We've had a few heated arguments here. It's been remarkable that we haven't had more perhaps because we've been selected as all being different. And as I said, just said now, I've never been on any group where I've been selected for being different. I've been on ones for selection for this or that but and we're all one group together. So it's not surprising. We've probably upset a few people between ourselves but we've come up with something at the end of it. And I think we're still remarkably cohesive, that's my view. Everyone else chip in if it's different. One thing has come up, this learning curve. We're just about getting to the point where we might be of use to you. If we get released for go with good conduct or whatever after one more meeting. We don't think we've been particularly productive. We would like you to look at that. Some people are suggesting a 25-year period but [laughter] you may, but certainly."

Man: "With a gold watch."

Harvey: "With a gold watch." [laughter] [talk continues]

A further common discursive style involved deliberating through the swapping or exchanging of stories of personal experiences. Extract 17 and Extract 18 below indicate how this worked. The first extract is from a small group session in the third meeting of the Council and the second from a small group discussion in the second meeting of the Council. Here the personal experiences recounted by Evelyn in Extract 17 and Bridget in Extract 18 become negotiable counters in the argument like pieces of evidence, and it is also a way of expressing or arguing a point of view. The exchange of these leads to a commonsense or life world position on what is reasonable through adducing stories and accounts of self and others' reactions.

Extract 17

David: "But the way it was put to us in Cardiff was that if somebody gets killed in a road accident at 20...."

Trudy: "Yeah."

David: "... you tend to feel 'oh what a shame he's missed out' but if my father dies at 80 it's natural. So that's what you know because he's had a fair innings."

Trudy: "... [inaudible] because he's a [inaudible] ..."

David: "Well because he's had a fair innings. Or someone gets killed in a road accident at 80, well he's had a fair innings so he was going to die sometime soon anyhow. So I'm not arguing the case I'm [multiple voices] ..."

[inaudible]

Evelyn: "Can I just add ..."

David: "That seems unfair to the 20-year-old because well he's missed out on his 60 years of life."

Evelyn: "Can I just have a personal view?"

Male: "Yeah."

Evelyn: "The thing is, now I lost my cousin at 39 in a road accident. Three or four years before that I lost my father who was 77. We felt a great deal more hurt and upset in a way through me cousin...."

Harry: "Cheated."

Evelyn: "... through because he ..."

Harry: "Sorry."

Evelyn: "... through me cousin."

Wendy: "Cheated, yes."

Evelyn: "Because of what he'd actually left behind. He'd got a young son and he kept going back to his flat. Well, he wanted to go and see."

Bridget: "I think that. You've got a potential future with that person."

Evelyn: [inaudible]

Bridget: "... of that future. He's been cheated out of that future [inaudible] in a way."

Extract 18

Fred: "I'd say the question of resuscitation. I'd like to know what their opinion on that is."

Bridget: "That's quite a good question because a year and a half ago my mum died and they actually called me into the consultant and said look. At the time she wasn't officially dying she was in hospital and they said 'if your mum's heart stops, or breathing, whatever do you want us to resuscitate her?'. We didn't even think about that and I was the first one asked of the family."

Wendy: "Mm."

Bridget: "And I decided to say no. I didn't want her resuscitated because in a way it's [inaudible] to me. Oh, you know, this is ... then just because she could suffer more if we resuscitate her. And my mother wasn't ready to die mentally at all, you know. But I agreed with them thinking now I was sort of in a way put under slight pressure the doctor liked me to go."

Fred: "Well, I have the same problem."

Female: "Yeah?"

Fred: "With my father. Like my father was 87 in hospital and they asked me that same question as well [inaudible] [background noise cough]. And I said yes [multiple voices] because ..."

Female: "... [inaudible] echoing [multiple voices] ..."

Bridget: "... [echoing] well my Mum [multiple voices] and she did have emphysema. But she didn't.... But, you know, they said she wasn't going to die. She wasn't totally worn out. She wasn't [inaudible] do you know what I mean? She wasn't elderly [multiple voices]...."

Fred: "See when everything closes down."

Female: "No, I'm sorry let's just ..."

Bridget: "Yes."

Female: "We've got that question now."

This account of some of the different discursive practices adopted by members of the Council is not intended to be exhaustive. Crucially, the fact that there were a variety of possible styles raises intriguing questions about the relations between different ways of talking. Were all the different discursive practices drawn on by members of the Council equal? Which became routine and which were censored?

Not all styles were equal. Some were more highly valued than others, and some ways of communicating became privileged as members of the Council policed themselves and each other to meet mostly implicit but widely shared standards of 'appropriate behaviour'. Some speakers, it seems, became constructed as rich in 'deliberative capital', while others became impoverished and lacking in such capital. Those seen as rich in such resources were listened to more attentively, became more influential in the group and were emulated, while those who were seen as lacking deliberative capital were marginalised and seen as behaving inappropriately. How did this work?

The valuing of the discursive practices that emerge in a deliberative assembly indicates the flow of power around and within the event. First, power in the group will, as critics of deliberation suggested, reflect social relations and external social divisions in society more generally. Not all the speaking styles members of a Council bring to the meeting will be equally valued *ab initio*. Speaking styles associated with different occupations, class positions and gender will come with a different value attached (Sanders, 1997; Barnes, 2002). This valuing is predictable, but can sometimes go against the direction of power relations in wider society. It was striking, for example, that one of the members of the NICE Citizens Council most highly valued by other members was a young male public sector worker who was particularly skilled at summary and debate. Indeed this member was informally elected as the leader or the Council spokesperson on a number of occasions in the first Council meeting. He resisted these pressures, and this role, as his own predilection was for more egalitarian interaction. The speech styles, on the other hand, brought by members of the Council from much more privileged social class backgrounds were not so automatically endorsed by the rest of the Council.

In addition to the patterns of social advantage and disadvantage embedded in the discursive practices brought to the Council there is the flow of power within the meeting itself – the forms of speaking which are validated on the day by powerful others, such as representatives of NICE, and which are supported by the institutional arrangements. As with the terms for inclusion discussed in the last section, the power relations circulating around a deliberative assembly are subtle. They have little to do with direct coercion and probably rarely involve the intentional strategic manipulation of others. Power is conveyed through what is taken for granted, what seems normal and natural, and the effects are subtle and emergent, often obvious only with hindsight.

In the NICE Citizens Council one of the most evident effects of this kind was the positioning that eventually emerged around personal narratives. As noted, use of personal narratives to make points was widespread. Indeed, 'telling a story' was a much more pervasive speech style than the three others considered earlier: the researcher, the adversarial and the chair of the committee. Over time, however, a tacit consensus emerged that some ways of doing personal anecdotes were acceptable and others were not. Deliberation based on the exchange of narratives to find a 'life world' response to an issue through the collection of personal examples became devalued.

The pattern around the censoring and sanctioning of the personal was complex. Some speakers were 'allowed' the personal and some were not. The devaluation of personal narratives was evident through informal comments to the chair, for example, that the facilitators should make sure "we keep on track and don't tell personal anecdotes". It was also evident in the hesitancy displayed by members of the Council in later meetings when they began to tell personal stories. They would frequently apologise in advance, present their example as a 'side issue', beg the Council's indulgence, and so on. And this hesitancy can be seen above in the way Evelyn introduces her story in Extract 17. The facilitators themselves made it clear that personal narratives were not always welcome. It became apparent relatively early to the members of the Council that the life world discourse of personal narrative was in conflict with the technical and professional discourse of the witnesses and NICE itself. These powerful and respected figures used a different kind of discourse, one based on reference to evidence, using generalisations, and inevitably they used a more complex vocabulary. Although the witnesses and representatives from NICE were invariably accommodating and polite in response to personal narratives, their bemusement at how to handle them, and the discourse used in the construction of the replies, conveyed a strong message about appropriate style. Perceiving this, the members of the Council adjusted their own discourse to fit. The 'researcher speech style' noted above, for example, was a product of this self-regulation.

Extracts 19 and 20 give two examples of the discursive clash. Extract 19 is taken from the opening session with the chair of NICE on the first day of the Cardiff meeting. The chair of NICE works hard to respond to Wendy's one-off example of a friend's experience and to bring the discussion back to the more general ground of regulations involving age. Wendy comes back, however, with a direct question asking for a personal response ("was he surprised?"), and he replies in that mode. Extract 20 is taken from a role-play in the third meeting in Sheffield, where councillors, facilitated by the appraisals programme director, worked as though they were an appraisal committee of NICE. Members of the Council again reason using the personal as a resource, and the director shifts the discourse back to the overall pattern of evidence.

In Chapter Five, material from this session with the programme director was considered as an example of how active facilitation could set a productive atmosphere for deliberation (see Extract 11 in Chapter Five), but now a particularly testing dilemma for the whole field of deliberative participation comes into sharper relief. Who gets to define what deliberation should look like, and is the deliberative ideal actually based on an implicit model of the university tutorial (see Chapter Two) rather than the ways in which citizens want to engage?

Extract 19

Facilitator: "Thank you Nick [laughing voice]. Wendy please."

Wendy: "I want to ask you does NICE have a policy about lower age limits for certain treatments. And I need to describe to you what I'm talking about before you answer me. A friend of mine, who's a similar age to me, who's got very bad arthritis in her knees (and so much so she's had to sell her house and get a bungalow because she can't manage the stairs). And she's been told at the hospital that she can't have knee replacement because she isn't old enough. Is that your policy?"

Chair: "No, no, I don't know where that came from, it is out of the ordinary...."

Wendy: "Well that's happened, actually happened."

Chair: "Yeah, well, it's off the wall, certainly people do something or other. We do have some difficulties though and I think they'll probably explore this, this afternoon. When these drugs go on the market they're often on the market regulated for a specific age group. When new drugs come on the market they're often not liberally tested on children. And if they are to be tested on the elderly, and we have to follow whatever the, err ,regulated authorities say about use in the children and use in the elderly, but that's not because we're being ageist, it's because the regulation authorities have not been satisfied that it is either safe or effective. In the elderly or the young it may look as if they're being ageist in some way. And sometimes we get accused of ageism. But, for example, there's a medicine called 'Ritalin' for hyperactive children and we recommended that it should be used but not in children under the age of five. And the reason why we said not in children under the age of five was because the regulators had not been satisfied with the safety with under fives. And so therefore it's not licensed by the regulating authority for the under fives. So we would [inaudible]. What the sort of regulation [inaudible] accused by the *Daily Mail*, not surprisingly, accused by the *Daily Mail* of denying this medicine to children [inaudible]."

Wendy: "So are you surprised then that people are getting told that there is a lower age limit for knee replacements?"

Chair: "I'm very surprised."

Wendy: "Right ..."

Chair: "I'm very surprised ..."

Extract 20
Director: "This is tricky."

Nigel: "I've actually [inaudible] been trying to get this drug for a year."

Director: "What [inaudible] the growth hormone?"

Nigel: "Yeah."

Alan: "Can you tell us what the question is again?"

Director: "Right, the question, the two things, because of course we're thinking about concentrating on age. So we've got two big issues. First is we've got children and we've got adults. Should we be viewing them differently?"

Male: "Yeah."

Director: "In terms of growth hormone treatment? So that's the first discussion forum. If we do [background noise] what do we need to do? So I'm just going to take some soundings on that first difference in difference between adults and children."

Joan: "Well, they have different needs."

Bridget: "Firstly I don't think, well I don't think you should do them differently in a way at the moment because quality of life. I suffer from a problem with my pituitary and you can feel absolutely awful. So I think most people would assume you mean definitely look at children as favourably and possibly not look at adults favourably."

Director: "Just so I'll take you back to the evidence [background noise] that [name] presented which shows a clear benefit for children in terms of how much they grow. And very much uncertainty about the benefits in adults 'cos of course we've got to be thinking about the evidence...."

Wendy: "Yeah."

Director: "... that's presented so any ..."

Bridget: "I've seen someone who's got a similar problem though I know what it feels like when you feel rotten."

Joan: "We know it well."

Bridget: "Mmm."

The kinds of disjuncture evident above between life world discourse made vivid through personal narratives and anecdotes and what we could call professional discourse seemed difficult for all concerned. Witnesses and representatives from NICE were in a quandary. Their expertise (and their 'capital' as a witness) depended on their mastery of evidence-based discourse, yet the members of the Council often requested a very different kind of interaction. For the members of the Council, they were there because they were 'not professional', yet this seems to be a situation where everyday ways of talking were not up to the job.

Church (1996) noted a similar clash and mutual incomprehension in her study of the inclusion of psychiatric survivors into a public consultation on community mental health in Canada. The more emotion-laden, personal and informal styles used by the psychiatric survivors were in conflict with the etiquette that was taken for granted by the committee. Again, as with diversity issues for the NICE Citizens Council, the clash became phrased by the committee as one of 'good manners' rather than a struggle over the definition of appropriate talk. Church describes also the 'psychological hegemony' (the phrase comes from Lyman, 1981) constructed by the committee and, for example, the covert rules about emotional expression that operated. There are some key differences, of course, between participation initiatives with relatively uninvolved citizens and consultations with patients likely to be directly affected by decisions, but in all participation exercises a set of tacit emotional rules for joining in is likely to emerge. This is a useful reminder that discursive styles are not just about ways of talking but construct ways of feeling and being.

Does the crowding out of personal narratives at some moments matter? Is it significant that the adversarial and other styles more associated with formal debate came to signify deliberative capital? Does it matter also that the Council tried to model the discursive practices of the experts (and the practices associated with debate and interviews on television), and used these to regulate their own conduct? These are issues that go far beyond the usual considerations involved in the design of deliberative initiatives. As many commentators have pointed out, the generalising, reasonable-seeming, evidence-based language of the professional middle-class expert is not a neutral *lingua franca* for political discussion. Here, it seems to invalidate a key form of testimony and contribution used by non-expert citizens. Yet the citizens' stories are highly relevant to the task they have been given of bringing their own perspectives to bear. Not to recognise their value in this context may be to miss a deliberative trick.

Our findings certainly put flesh on Iris Young's (2000) concern that the discursive styles of the privileged and the powerful will dominate deliberative assemblies. Here capture is not necessarily a matter of content (of the viewpoints being argued). No one is suggesting that the Citizens councillors were cynically subverted. But since the discursive practices people use also carry their world views and values, there is also much more at stake than simple issues of presentation. A few of the members of the Council had access, if not quite to the expert style, to comparable authoritative styles; many did not, however. In most deliberative initiatives, active effort will need to be put into identifying, validating and celebrating other ways of speaking and unpacking the discursive logics.

Identities, positions and frames: the 'extraordinarily ordinary' citizen

> I assume that definitions of a situation are built up in accordance with principles of organization which govern events [...] and our subjective involvement in them; frame is the word I use to refer to such of these basic elements as I am able to identify. (Goffman, 1974: 10)

Participants bring their pre-existing social identities with them to a new community of practice, such as their ethnic group membership, their status as a young or older person, their gender and so on, and these identities become worked up as speaking positions and signified afresh in this new context. Deliberative initiatives, however, also seem to demand some further, in some ways more puzzling, forms of identity work – those associated with the position of the citizen itself. Indeed, what kind of identity could this be – the 'extraordinarily ordinary citizen', as members were described in the course of the first Council meeting? Particularly in the first Citizens Council meeting this was a pressing puzzle for the members of the Council – why were they there and what could they contribute?

> **Extract 21**
>
> Graham: "Do you, do you expect us to come up with something radically different to what medical professionals have already done because medical professionals [inaudible] in teams as well. Y'know, you've got the sea of prejudices that your [inaudible] group has, you've got in this room. Are you expecting us to come up with something different or do you think that there is something about health professionals that biases them one way?"
>
> Chair of NICE: "Well, I don't, I don't know. I mean I was actually won—
> ... thinking that [inaudible] whether your views are very different to th— to, to mine. But one of the problems in health professionals – they'll kill me now for saying this – erm, is th—, that health professionals tend to be terribly blinkered. Erm, if you're a heart surgeon, everything is heart surgery. And you, you just shut your eyes to all the other needs of the, of the health service. You are concentrating on that, erm, and to the exclusion almost of everything else. And, and doctors also by their training are expected to concentrate on the needs of individual patients in (inaudible) and not worrying about anyone else."
>
> [...]
>
> Graham: "So you are expecting us to see the whole picture?"
>
> Chair: "We're asking you to see the whole picture rather than [inaudible] ..."

In this very early exchange in the first Citizens Council meeting one relatively firm answer emerges – what a citizen does is to 'see the whole picture'. Other similar answers also quickly emerged. The citizen is disinterested, impartial and unbiased compared to the interested expert or lobbyist. The citizen is also typically 'down to earth' while the health professional or academic engages in ivory tower mystification. The citizen possesses common sense as opposed to abstruse rationality.

These local, for the event, constructions of citizen identities were closely related to two dominant frames (in Goffman's sense of the term) which emerged in the course of the NICE Citizens Council. One of these frames was 'interrogation' and the other was 'education'. The frame of interrogation was already set up by the terminology of 'juries' and 'witnesses'. The citizen's role was to interrogate the expert witness and indeed put them on the defensive – "give them a grilling", as one facilitator exhorted. The 'down to earth', 'disinterested', 'seeing the whole picture' citizen becomes a watchdog in this frame, sniffing out the actuality behind the obfuscating words of the expert, on behalf of all citizens everywhere. Extract 22, below, illustrates this adversarial or interrogatory style. The extract is taken from the first meeting of the Council and from the question session with a witness from the pharmaceutical industry.

Extract 22

Facilitator: "Okay, that is great. Let's see. Alan, were you indicating with a question?"

Alan: "Hello, doctor."

Facilitator: "And then Graham after that, and then Wendy."

ABPI director: "[name] please." [witness asks to be called by his first name]

Alan: "Hello [name]. [name], don't you think that it is morally wrong that a drug company should pass on the costs of all their failed experiments and tests on the drugs that do work, especially onto the NHS? If I was to do a job at your house, I am a [description of the speaker's job given at this point], if I was to do a job at your house I wouldn't expect you to pay for a job I had failed on further down the street."

ABPI director: "That is a very, very, good question. The fact is though that in order for there to be any further research and development then you have to make profit in order to be able to push that back in, into research and development...."

This watchdog or adversarial relationship between the expert and the citizen sits uneasily and uncomfortably, however, with the concept of the Citizens Council as an advisory body, adding a citizen's view on the values which should inform NICE decision making. Bodies advising on values and watchdogs scrutinising actions and policies are very different frames indeed. And some of this contradiction goes back to the early confusions in NICE itself, discussed in Chapter Three, about the purpose of the Citizens Council. This discrepancy reflects the mismatch which can occur when technologies like the citizens' jury design are applied regardless of whether the framing and rhetoric of the jury and the identity positions it supplies are appropriate for the deliberative context and objective.

The second dominant frame of 'education' set up by the NICE Citizens Council came from the emphasis in the design and organisation of events on 'informing citizens'. The relatively powerful watchdog position for the citizen thus alternated with a much less powerful 'deficit' position of the student in a tutorial. The witness was the expert, and the member of the Council was the student trying to learn from them. When questioning in this frame, members of the Council tended to defer to witnesses. This deference was reinforced by the nature of the witnesses chosen for the Council. These were often highly successful individuals selected through NICE's own extensive networks. Both NICE and Vision 21 had worked hard to get those they felt were the best speakers and most authoritative and knowledgeable representatives of different perspectives and stakeholder groups in the field. The members of the Council often commented at how impressed they were by the witnesses, and grateful to have the opportunity to listen to them. "It is not every day," one noted, "you get the undivided attention of an NHS consultant". But while it may have been interesting to hear from such high quality witnesses, it only increased the puzzle about what the 'ordinary citizen' could offer and their authority to express any opinion at all.

The citizens seemed to be caught then between the necessity of learning to do their job and the struggle to find some more powerful and autonomous position to confront the expert on more equal terms. This was an intense contradiction. 'Becoming informed' by experts implied that the citizen was in the 'down position', yet a deliberative forum was precisely the situation in which the citizen was to be king, would have the last word, and should be listened to. Being a watchdog wasn't the answer because that wasn't really the brief. Yet what other expertise could the citizen muster to take charge here? What kind of expertise does, for example, being 'down to earth' and 'disinterested' translate into?

In practice the councillors resolved this dilemma by alternating between being 'students' and acting out implicit and sometimes very explicit resistance to the professionals and experts. This resistance took a number of forms, overvaluing, for instance, the words and testimony of those witnesses who were identifiably less or non-expert (such as patients, nurses, carers and front-line workers). It included contempt for those experts who didn't seem to have any hands-on experience. The citizens occasionally would become the *enfant terrible* in the proceedings, the child who had to be deferred to and could behave badly because that was what they seemed to be there for: to attack and evaluate, rather than suggest new creative routes. The onus was put on the expert to formulate and work things out and to take responsibility. One of the ideals behind deliberation, however, is that it goes beyond critique to find new and better solutions.

In raising these questions of identity positions and frames we are pointing to some wider issues for any deliberative assembly. Bang and Dryberg (2000), for example, have argued that deliberation depends on the negotiation of a relationship of co-governance between citizen and expert. As we noted in Chapter Two, this is the view that deliberation rests on a candid acceptance of the differences between experts and citizens and their joint responsibilities. Co-governance implies, however, that these questions about the expertise and role of the citizen will have received careful thought and attention, and that there is a lot more clarity about what the citizen brings to the table.

The second, closely related, point is simply to note what the introduction of the lay–expert binary into the proceedings does. The requirement that citizens 'become informed' potentially undercuts the aim of deliberation to strengthen and extend democracy. Identity is always defined relationally, through otherness, contrast and comparison. The powerful and highly salient binary categorisation of lay versus expert inevitably fills out, configures and constructs the cultural and political identity slot of 'the citizen' in some highly specific ways. Sustained consideration needs to be given to how one can be a citizen when there are experts around, and this needs active discussion as part of the ground rules for the event.

Finally, it is worth noting that there are many ways in which a citizen identity could be defined within a democracy and there has been, of course, extensive political debate about what the term 'citizen' signifies. Some of these constructions of citizen identity are more empowering than others. Worryingly, the identity of the down-to-earth, commonsense, disinterested adjudicator citizen does not seem to be a sufficient foundation for building a collective citizen view. A community of practice like the Citizens Council becomes defined simply as a collective of the sensible. All the councillors come to have in common is their difference from the experts, marginalising any of the other interests and priorities a collective group of citizens might have in a democratic deliberation. It is difficult to organise a coherent response or 'do democratic politics' on the basis of being down to earth alone. As Hogg and Williamson (2001: 4) have argued, the legendary 'wise fool', possessing nothing but common sense, is an ambiguous and precarious basis for democratic participation. In contrast to the expert, the citizen has just personal experience as their authority to speak. They are thrown back, therefore, on just the points of greatest division among them – their idiosyncratic life experiences – that can prove very difficult to coordinate into a consensual worked-out response to the question asked.

Conclusion

This chapter has documented a number of ways in which power can swirl around the arena of a deliberative assembly creating contradictions and dilemmas. Power is there in the way knowledge is constructed; it is there in the dominance of the voice and perspective of the white ethnic majority and the terms that are set for minority group participation. It is there, too, in the delicate accommodations reached between different possible discursive styles for deliberating, and in the clash between the evidence-based discourse of the professional and the personal narratives of the councillors. Finally, power is there in the whole way the scene is set, in the very notion of 'becoming informed' and the lay–expert divide. The citizen identity in this case became defined as an attitude of commonsense scepticism leading to questions about whether 'ordinariness' can be a sufficiently substantive and empowering group identity for participation and democratic deliberation. Whether these various effects of power invalidate the ideal of deliberation is a difficult issue to which we will return in Part III.

What is worth noting here is that the construction of an adequate 'expertise space' for the citizen participant is more than a matter of the issues raised in previous chapters about design, modes of engagement, types of witnesses and styles of facilitation. In this chapter we have multiplied the points that a convenor of a deliberative forum needs to consider. These include the ways in which citizens are invited in and addressed, which discursive styles are supported and reinforced, and how these interact with the norms and prescriptions for good deliberation. Should citizens be trained in how to deliberate or is that to miss the point of citizen participation? There is also the question of how a democratic space depends on non-democratically instituted ground rules and where the boundaries lie. The value of what citizens can offer will depend crucially on the kind of expertise space that is put together. However, value also depends on how the citizens' contributions are subsequently used and assessed. The next chapter looks at the reception of the material from the NICE Citizens Council as the ball returned to the Institute, and shows that the process of construction continues.

SEVEN

Reactions, reflections and reworkings

> Public participation is an activity that encompasses much
> more than the actual meeting period. Each participation
> project has a history and is followed by social and political
> repercussions. (Renn et al, 1995: 362)

It is clear that over the first two and a half years of the Citizens
Council initiative, the Institute put a great deal of time into shaping
just how the Council should work and into modifying its decisions
in the light of experience. We have argued that the changes served
to create more of an expertise space for citizens and that there was
a perceptible rise in the amount of deliberation; we have also shown
that important challenges remained. This chapter, the final one in
the series presenting empirical data, will explore the thinking that
accompanied change within the host organisation. The discursive
turn in the study of organisations is particularly helpful here, in its
insistence that talk in organisations is not a mere prelude or
preliminary to action; instead it much more actively creates and
constructs action (Weick, 2004). Chapter Three has already
demonstrated how, in setting up the Citizens Council, key players
within NICE rehearsed and reframed what were potentially hostile
stakeholder constructions of the Institute, placing this latest
innovation within their own emerging narratives of the significance
of the organisation and its mode of operation. This meaning making
continued and intensified as the dynamics of the development of
the Council began to unfold. A council fit for citizens had also to
be a council fit for purpose within the Institute, and it had to be
seen to be so among the different stakeholders to whom NICE
related. This chapter traces the discursive work of reframing, and
sometimes work of repair, in the face of real and imagined forms of
stakeholder interrogation and challenge.

The analysis proceeds via an examination of three particular
moments in the overall period under study, each a moment of
intense dialogic exchange about the emergent practice that was the

Citizens Council. The first section focuses on the aftermath of the first meeting, as the steering committee received the Council's first report and heard the ways in which the facilitators, the project manager and others themselves reconstructed their experiences of the meeting. Which interpretations were relinquished at this point, and which ones remained? The second section traces the ways in which different stakeholders, internal and external, intervened to assess the value of the Council. As staff within the Institute had anticipated, 'value for money' questions were one recurring theme. Other issues began to open up around the capacity of citizens, the quality of their deliberations and the degree of power that was granted to them by the Institute. The chapter focuses the most attention (in the third section) on the point, two years on, when a series of workshops was convened to explore the potential use of Council reports. This brought the Institute's programme directors more firmly into the debate than hitherto, and served to open up the question of whether it was not time to overturn the 'working at one remove' and 'dealing with a meta-question' strategies outlined in Chapter Three. The debate also brought members of the Institute's advisory committees into the picture. Drawn from the wider academic and practice community, they serve as a vitally important resource in the development of appraisals and guidelines and in the creation of legitimacy for the evidence base that feeds into NICE guidelines. Echoing some of the critics of the deliberative ideal discussed in Chapter Two, these interrogations underlined the different directions from which queries could emerge, and the multiple ways in which deliberation itself could be construed as a contested and contestable practice.

The major sources for this chapter are the detailed field notes compiled from observation of meetings of the steering committee, board meetings and other occasions where the Citizens Council was discussed. The analytical strategy, focusing in on three particular moments, serves two purposes. First, it provides a means by which we are able to enter imaginatively into worldviews in the host organisation, to give a flavour of the dilemmas that a participatory initiative generates, and to trace the handling of these through repeated sense-making efforts carried out with and for audiences whose legitimation for the exercise is sought. Second, seen in the context of the preceding chapters, this analysis begins to reveal what might be theorised as a clash of two communities of practice – that which was emerging in the Citizens Council and that of the Institute itself. In doing so, it points to the need to develop and embellish the theoretical framework with which this study has worked. This will be taken up in Part III. Box 7.1 lists, in sequence, the key events that are discussed in this chapter, linking them with the dates of meetings of the Council. It thus serves to help keep the chronology in view. All the Citizens Council reports discussed in this chapter are available for public scrutiny and have been posted under the relevant section of the NICE website (see www.nice.org.uk).

Box 7.1: Some key events

2002

November Induction weekend for Council members

November First Citizens Council meeting – discusses 'clinical need'

December First report on website

2003

January NICE board discusses first report

January/March Two internal topic-setting workshops re 'age'

March NICE Partners Council discusses the Council and the first report

May Second Citizens Council meeting – interim discussion on age

July NICE board discusses second report

September In-house circulation of 'Scientific and social value judgements'

October Parliamentary reception for Council members

November Third Citizens Council meeting – final age report

2004

January NICE board discusses third report (final age report)

2004 (contd)

May Fourth Citizens Council report – confidential enquiries

June/July Four impact workshops take place

July NICE board meeting discusses fourth report

A first review of product and process

Two weeks after the Citizens Council's first meeting (in December 2002), staff from the Institute's programmes were invited to join the steering committee in receiving the report from the Citizens Council. First-hand experience of the Council varied among the group present. The facilitators, who were now in attendance, had had the closest contact; they had also authored the report. The project manager had observed the whole of the first Council meeting, intervening at times to clarify. The chair, chief executive and directors of the three programmes had given presentations, and arriving early for these or leaving late gave them more of a flavour of what had happened. The video-recordings and transcripts from the research project and our analyses of these, at this point, were very much in the future.

The facilitators constructed events in an upbeat way. They had engaged in much hard work behind the scenes in supporting and reassuring Council members as well as being on stage throughout. As one of the facilitation team was later to put it:

> "Everything worked! The hotel was very good, easier than the one we had used for the Induction.... It was very demanding being at the beck and call of 30 people. And very long hours: from 8.30 am to after dinner writing up the notes. The best thing was that at the beginning when people were asking 'how can we do this?' – and we did! The main thing is how nice the Council members were – a nice bunch of people, and you thought about its impact on people's lives."

Two senior staff from NICE who had attended part of the meeting on the second day as expert witnesses and also observed some other witness sessions had more mixed perceptions. One stated firmly that:

"It was clear that they understood what we were doing by the end of the session, and they seemed very committed and engaged. I came away feeling positive.... They were thirsty to know things."

Another, however, who had had the opportunity to watch the proceedings in much the same way, expressed some doubt, commenting that Council members did not seem to know the appropriate questions for each witness. These problems, ones as we have seen that were later to be revealed more systematically from the evidence of the observation study, were understandably perhaps underplayed, in face of much that had gone well.

The group heard an account of the 'quiet revolt' when Council members 'threw out' the facilitators and the observers and held a session on their own. This whole episode became framed in subsequent discussions in steering committee meetings and elsewhere as an iconic anecdote which presented the Citizens Council as strong and independent-minded people, who were not under anyone's sway: vindication, that is, of the 'no capture, no contamination' aim. The facilitators, however, commented that such an incident was 'business as usual': "in every single citizens' jury we have done we've been thrown out – and asked back in!". More important at this point, however, was the matter of the first report of the Citizens Council and its contents.

Participants had gathered round a large table, each with their copy of the report. This was 25 pages long, in very large print, with bullet point lists and each section starting on a fresh page. It began with an executive summary of the factors that the Council had considered most important in relation to 'clinical need'. These were then presented in more detail, framed as the answers to the set of questions posed. The phrase 'in no specific order' recurred throughout. The report ended with recommendations. These included recommendations concerning the organisation of the Council itself – criticisms of the 'retirement' policy, for example, and a call for advance notice of the topic.

As the assembled group started to discuss the report, unease began to mount. There was puzzlement over seeming internal inconsistencies in the document, and someone suggested that perhaps an 'independent editor' should be brought in to help. It was argued, however, that since this was the Citizens Council's own report, making editorial suggestions would not be appropriate. Dissatisfaction was expressed about the absence of ranking and weighting, mostly by staff from the appraisals and guidelines programmes, who found that, without this, the report did not provide them with very much of substance to work with. Questions were asked as to exactly how Council members' views had been translated into the report. The facilitators described a 'ghost-writing' process, conducted at speed following the Council meeting, while memories were still fresh. Copious notes were assembled into a first draft, Council members responded voluminously, and the final draft sought conscientiously to accommodate all comments before being sent out to members again. At this point, "we took silence for consent". The report, like the facilitation of the meetings, reflected a strong concern with inclusivity. This assembly of opinions and ideas was proving difficult to interpret, let alone to operationalise.

Focusing on the report-writing process was perhaps an easy target. The difficulty of understanding the topic and task, the absence of deliberation and the nature of the review sessions (see Chapter Four) were inevitably going to give the facilitators a headache as far as report preparation was concerned. Steering committee members, however, reassured each other: "we aren't expecting answers in a day – but to start the process". And in default of finding much direct enlightenment on the subject of clinical need, the group turned to the Council's procedural suggestions, which seemed more straightforward. They restated the principle that the Council should be 'refreshed', but in a spirit of compromise, responded to dissatisfaction with the 'retirement policy' by agreeing that three meetings rather than two was acceptable, although a full three years was not. They also felt able to agree with the suggestion that the topic should be sent out to Council members in advance, and with the idea that the Council should have a say in calling witnesses.

By the end of a long meeting, it had been accepted that the Institute would need to engage with the Council about some of the puzzling or inconsistent things in the report, and in particular the enigmatic claim that 'age should be taken into consideration' would be a good topic to investigate further. A subsequent subgroup of the steering committee confirmed 'age' as the topic for the next Council meeting. In practice, each of the Council's three reports during the period of our study produced an adjustment on design. The first report on clinical need led to the selection of the topic of age and produced a two-meeting model. The second report on age led to the idea of including different approaches in consulting the public (discussed later in the chapter). And the third report on confidential enquiries led to a new format for the report, with a clearer acknowledgement of minority views and graphic demonstration of how people had changed their minds.

At this time, however, such changes were well in the future. In the course of this discussion, both the facilitators and the project manager had fed back to the steering committee a sense of the struggle that Citizens Council members had had with the question and the topic. Interviews with NICE staff (carried out shortly after the Council had deliberated on the question of 'clinical need', but before they had had the chance to read the report), acknowledged a problem. "We distilled the 'clinical need' question rather clumsily," said one; another felt with hindsight that "we were not thinking about how to present these issues to lay folk". Significantly, however, *speed* was identified as the main culprit – the Institute, it was felt, had just not spent enough time working on setting the topic.

The procedures that had led to the framing of 'clinical need' as the first question were again put in train. A topic-setting workshop was convened in March 2003 to explore 'age' as the theme for the second and third Council meetings. Detailed observation notes from this event demonstrate how eagerly the most senior staff in the Institute availed themselves of the opportunity to discuss the social value judgements that pervaded their work on the various NICE committees. Coffee and biscuits were left ignored, as participants' enthusiasm for sharing anecdotes and dilemmas proved sufficient to sustain them for a whole morning. As with accounts given to the research team of the two topic-setting workshops that had preceded the first meeting of the Council, insiders were once again seizing the opportunity to discuss values and to reflect on the complexity of the task of the Institute. Absent from the discussion, however, was just how to translate this into a question suitable for an outsider group to tackle. Participants were skilled in imagining and rehearsing the social constructions of NICE from the more immediate array of external stakeholders with which they were surrounded (see Chapter Three). They were not, it seemed, at this point imaginatively entering the world of the 'ordinary citizen' and framing a question that would elicit a confident response. Trouble with the question was to pervade both meetings on age. "I don't understand what they don't understand," the chief executive was observed to comment at one point, a comment accompanied by an audible sigh of frustration.

How might one sum up? In terms of aligning the emerging community of practice that was the Citizens Council with the more established one of the Institute, this set of events was particularly revealing. Different ways of conducting the Council meetings had begun to open up (fewer witnesses, for example, and more role-play); but attachments to the strategies of keeping the Council at one remove from the day-to-day work, and of asking a meta-question were still intact. The gulf between the worlds inhabited by NICE, and the worlds of the citizens on the Council had narrowed, but still remained.

Whatever the internal discussions, a coherent account was needed for the outside world. How would the Institute's varied stakeholders receive the first fruits of the Council? The next section follows the first report from this point onto the website and into the meeting of the board. It draws on observations at the points where board meetings considered the first reports, and also considers reactions from the Partners Council.

Engaging directly with stakeholders

The Citizens Council reports were the most tangible products of the Council, visible to both the staff and networks of the Institute and to the outside world. They would become the medium through which the Institute would be judged in its translation of the idea of a Council into practice. Normal procedure for NICE is to place draft documents on its website, and also to send them directly to important stakeholders. There was concern, however, about what people would make of this first report, including doubts about how members of the Institute's advisory committees would react to receiving it 'cold'. After much debate, it was decided to put the report on the website with an accompanying press release, as well as sending copies to board members and the Department of Health. Following discussion at the NICE board in January 2003, the Institute's formal response would be sent out to stakeholders and then placed on the web. It was felt that enhancing the Council's role in the public domain was important, and positive press attention would be useful.

'NICE Citizens Council issues first "common sense" report' was the headline on the Institute's website on 20 December 2002. Comments were invited. Possibly due to the imminent approach of Christmas and the concentration of the media on the approaching international conflict in Iraq, no web responses were received. However, in addition to formal acknowledgements from the Secretary of State and the Royal College of Nursing, NICE received written comments from both Help the Aged and from their own group Patients Involved in NICE (PIN), as well as reports of comments made by the retiring head of the Alzheimer's Society at a conference. The comments all focused on the reference in the report to age as a factor 'to be taken into consideration' when considering clinical need. All were negative. These reactions were among the factors pushing the subject of 'age' up the steering committee's agenda (see below).

Board meetings were a public site of dialogue, where stakeholders had an opportunity to interrogate the Institute, to construct and reconstruct understandings of the Council. Some of those internal to NICE but less directly involved were part of this, as were Citizens Council members themselves. Two Council members (supported by a facilitator) presented the first report to the board at its meeting in January 2003, answering questions both from members of the board and from the public present. When Evelyn introduced the report, she chose to stress how "un-influenceable" by NICE the Citizens Council was. Martin, meanwhile, added that he was pleased to read in the board's formal response to the report that they had recognised the Council's points. He repeated that Council members wanted more time to discuss various issues at future meetings, and emphasised the strong challenge that Council members had made to the retirement policy. Both Evelyn and Martin reported that they had faced "a steep learning curve", but found it both interesting and worthwhile.

Presenting their second report to a board meeting, two other Council members were more critical of the intelligibility of the questions put to them:

> "If we could understand how NICE developed the question, that would help us ... we need to know why you want to know...." (Graham)

> "We want the ... question re-phrased – so we can understand it better!" (Rachael)

Returning to the board's formal response to the first report, requests for procedural change – a three-meeting tenure, advance notice of topic, and some say in witness selection – were accepted in principle, as were aspects of the substantive points. The board responded to the Council's recommendation that NICE advisory bodies should 'take into account' the question of the age of the patient by batting the issue back:

> "It is unclear from the Council's report in what way they think the Institute and its advisors should do this. As a consequence, the board considers that this issue should

be the subject of further consideration by the Council at an early future meeting."

The issue now arose as to what the status of the Citizens Council report was to be. The chief executive announced an intention to publish a formal policy document, binding on all the Institute's advisory committees, within a year. It would be 'a living document', continually evolving in the light of future Council reports. One of the non-executive board members, however, raised the 'hierarchy of evidence' issue: how did the Citizens Council report fit with other evidence that might be available on the values and priorities of the public? Discussion was limited, but later this point was to puzzle members of the advisory committees and lead to more extended challenges.

Costs were probably always going to be a factor. Table 7.1 shows a detailed costs breakdown covering the induction event and first three Council meetings, prepared at the request of the research team. Even without factoring in the time of the steering committee members and senior staff, the cost per meeting was well in excess of £100,000. Running a national-level, residential event is a much more costly business than, say, a local authority's citizens' jury involving residents. Local juries, it has been suggested recently, average at around £25,000 (Parkinson, 2004b).

Table 7.1: Citizens Council costs (2002-04)

Recruitment of Council members[1]	£72,731
Council member fees[2]	£62,000
Third party agency (Vision 21)[3]	£142,935
Travel expenses[4]	£10,000
Venue costs[5]	£57,000
Institute support staff[6]	£101,551
Children and Young People Project[7]	£23,500
Total	**£469,717**

Notes:

[1] Includes national advertising and fees to the agency handling the recruitment process.

[2] Includes attendance for 30 members at induction and three meetings, plus some initial media training for a subset of some members.

[3] Includes costs of facilitating induction and three meetings and preparing reports.

[4] In addition to Council members, includes the costs of Institute staff, witnesses and the evaluation team.

[5] Covers costs of four residential meetings in a spread of locations in England and Wales.

[6] Includes a full-time project manager for the majority of this time.

[7] Costs of securing additional information on age from a project facilitated by the NCB.

At the board meeting considering the first report, a suggestion that in-house facilitation would be cheaper was energetically rebutted. Questions about value for money recurred whenever the Citizens Council was on the agenda – asked by non-executive members of the board as well as by members of the public. "Would you pay fifty grand for that report?", someone was heard to mutter on their way out of one such meeting. Value for money was never far below the surface for any of the participants. Individual members of the Council themselves sometimes queried the usefulness of what they were doing, and whether or not they were just a 'cosmetic exercise'. The chief executive and the chair spoke in several steering committee meetings about their concern with being able to show that the not inconsiderable sums of money spent on the Council had in fact been an investment in the ongoing search for better decision-making processes within the Institute. The fact that in 2004 NICE became directly responsible to Parliament and therefore to the Public Accounts Committee no doubt helped to concentrate minds.

Another key site for dialogue about the nature of the Council and its value was the Partners Council. We have already noted the diverse critics represented on this large body meeting three times a year, and the power of organised patient groups on it. It was not lost on this body that the line in the NHS Plan unveiling the Citizens Council had ambiguities and seemed not to acknowledge the growing role of patients and patient groups in the processes of NICE. The head of the NHS Strategy Unit had been invited early on to address a meeting of the Partners Council and to discuss their concerns. The chair doubtless had this experience in mind in addressing the Partners Council in March 2003. He gave a brisk run-through of all the stages to date, recruitment, induction, first meeting and report, dwelling in particular on the independence of the Council. The induction was portrayed as "one of the most vigorous cross-examinations we have ever had"; Citizens Council members were claimed as certainly "not shrinking violets". As to the first meeting, he said: "Don't expect an easy ride. They threw the facilitators out and it was 20 minutes before they needed the facilitators back". Left on the screen behind him as the discussion opened was a quotation that had come to his attention from Thomas Jefferson – about informing the people and trusting them to come to a wise decision.

The questions that followed focused on power and potential capture. These were dangers all too well known to those in this audience who worked in service user and carer organisations. The first questioner objected that NICE was both setting the question and deciding on the witnesses. The chair responded:

> "They must be questions we need answers to and are prepared to act on. For example, we thought about asking about the hierarchy of evidence – RCTs to anecdotes – we couldn't use the answer if it were that anecdotes are more important."

This served to open up the discussion further. Just how far could scientific judgements and value judgements be distinguished? Did 'trust the people' not imply that 'you can empower the people to tackle any question'? The matter was closed in a joking way. "We are not a university," observed the deputy chair, and the chair himself laughingly mused "perhaps we should bring Iain Chalmers [a prominent epidemiologist, well known to the audience] in". The agenda for the meeting was full and a particularly important issue for the service representatives present was next – a discussion of how the consultation on changes to the appraisal process was going to be handled. By the end of the discussion of the Citizens Council, the top table had given way on some points – welcoming comments about the questions to be set and accepting the recommendation that the Partners Council may well have suggestions as to names of witnesses to be called. It was clear, however, that the Citizens Council was not a topic that would go through Partners Council meetings on the nod.

Public exchanges about the value of the Citizens Council at board meetings and the Partners Council reveal a number of points. First, they demonstrate the continued commitment of the Institute to transparency and openness – a key part of the organisational narrative. Second, not everything was anticipated in the operating model. Board meetings showed participants thinking on their feet about the complicated issue of 'the join' between the process and the product and how to use the reports. Third, the value for money issue, always in the minds of participants, was emerging as predicted. Fourth, complex questions about the kinds of evidence represented by the reports were entangled with all this. This was to become more prominent as the next section now reveals. Already, however, it is clear that sites of public debate figure prominently in prompted constructions and reconstructions of the significance of the Citizens Council.

Questions of role and status

With discussions of the first report behind them, senior staff in the Institute gave attention to formulating the next question for the Council, and to how to redesign a deliberative event. They also began to express growing concern about how much credence could and should be placed on its pronouncements and to where exactly its decisions should sit within the policies and procedures of NICE.

The chair and vice-chair of the Institute (both members of the Citizens Council steering committee) began work on a 'values paper'. Following a long gestation period, a draft was circulated in-house in September 2003. The document was entitled 'Scientific and social value judgements'. It took an overarching and integrative position, explaining that it now emerged as a result of the whole gamut of experience of the Institute:

> This document is intended to be used as a point of reference by those responsible for developing the Institute's guidance, as well as a source of information for those who are interested in NICE's work. It is based on the experience of its advisory committees, appeal panels, national collaborating centres and guideline development groups. It has also been informed by the deliberations of its Citizens Council. (Rawlins and Culyer, 2003: App 5)

That last line was acknowledgement of the concern that Council members should be able to see a concrete product to which their work had contributed. It was the first official document of the Institute to recognise the input of the Citizens Council.

The document acknowledged that social value judgements lurk within 'clinical effectiveness' and 'cost'; it made a firm distinction between the two as used by the Institute in its work and accepted that both had a role to play. This was not new. It went on, however, to take the position that, in advising the NHS, "the Institute should embody values that are generally held by those that the NHS serves" (ibid). The phrase about 'values generally held' was particularly telling, and one to which we shall return. In consequence, the paper continued, the Institute was not only committed to developing the Citizens Council, but also to commissioning *other research* to identify the views of the public. Where did this leave the Citizens Council and its reports? In practice, the answer was not very clear.

The Citizens Council had moved from the enigmatic 'age as a factor' position in their first report, to age as something that should *not* be taken into account in their second. Overall, the steering committee was much happier with this, the interim report on age, than with the report on clinical need, but they found this conclusion surprising. At the board meeting, the chief executive felt moved to confirm this with the Council representatives present. Had they really meant that "just because kids are kids the NHS doesn't have to be more generous to them"? Their reply was clear: "We thought one year of life was equally valid at any age. But we do tend to think differently when it's our own children!".

The steering committee decided that this needed more testing. They therefore bought space in an ICM Omnibus poll to include questions on age. Results were available at their next meeting (May 2003). These results were at variance with the position of the Council. Some now seized on the idea of polling; at a cost of around £6,000, it would save money and be "a wonderfully efficient operation – all in a week". Others argued to the contrary, that it was proof of the value of using a deliberative method rather than a snapshot of 'gut reactions':

> "This [survey] justifies the Citizens Council; polling doesn't pick up on things like the Council does."

> "The whole point of having a deliberative Council is shown by the way people prioritised by age and social role in the poll."

Still others were more sceptical, observing that since research was the business of NICE, they should not be accepting as justification a completely different piece of work, using different questions asked in a different context (a telephone survey):

> "It looks as if NICE is setting one set of evidential standards for its guidance, and another wishy-washy one for this."

From this point, the committee became increasingly interested in exploring different methods of accessing the views of the public. This eventually resulted in plans, as they were to put it, to 'triangulate' the responses to questions set for the Council at subsequent meetings, by simultaneously commissioning a poll and focus groups.

In the summer of 2004, four impact workshops were held, the primary aim of which was to explore potential uses for the Citizens Council reports. The workshops constituted an arena in which staff from the appraisals and guidelines programmes and their external advisory group members were given the time and opportunity to reflect on their work and the difficult judgements it involved. This was reminiscent of the topic-setting workshops for the Council. The workshops also served to stimulate steering committee members into fresh and intense episodes of sense making – formulating new elaboration of their own narratives about the rationale for the Council and its placement.

The format for all four workshops was much the same: initial presentations about the Council by the project manager, the clinical director or the director of planning and resources, and by the facilitators, a question-and-answer session, followed by small group discussions and finally a plenary session. There was considerable strategic-level commitment to these workshops. The non-executives on the steering committee were invited to be facilitators of the small groups, and the plenary sessions were to be chaired respectively by the chairs of the appraisals committees, the clinical director, the guidelines programme director, and the director of planning and resources. The chair of the Institute cancelled other engagements in order to be present at some of these, thereby demonstrating his commitment to ensuring that the Citizens Council outputs would be used within the Institute.

The ways in which the steering committee members formulated and presented their own evolving conceptualisations of the Council from the perspective of two and a half years into the project demonstrated the legacy of initial perspectives. Addressing the question 'Why a Citizens Council?', the project manager emphasised two things: the Institute's desire for a 'standing' council, analogous to the Partners Council, rather than a one-off citizens' jury; and the importance of a deliberative body: "We want to know what decisions they make, and why, and how. The deliberative nature of the Citizens Council is very important". The facilitator's presentation extended this line of argument by pointing out that it was a 'council' and not a 'jury' because it was about values and not about reaching a verdict. "It is not a decision-making body." Council members, she said, were "challenged to know their own minds better".

The clinical director (who also had responsibility for the Research and Development [R&D] Programme within NICE) framed the Council as part of a wider ongoing research programme exploring societal values with regard to health gains. He now presented the Council as one among several NHS R&D projects working in the same area, others being conducted by health economists on the societal value of health gains and the value of the QALY (quality-adjusted life year). He also pointed with approval to the steering committee's plan for 'triangulation' of different methods for ascertaining the views of the public (polling, focus groups) for future Council meetings. Seemingly counter-intuitive results on age and on self-induced illness (where the Council's first report had indicated that this should not be a criterion for refusal to treat), had led him in this direction.

The first appraisals workshop had the biggest attendance. The members of the appraisals committees present had all been sent documents in advance relating to the Citizens Council, including its two first reports. From subsequent discussions and questions it was clear that most people had read them diligently and with interest; it was also clear that they had had little knowledge of the Council before this. The questions from the floor were wide-ranging and challenging. Participants were concerned about the status of the Council as an authoritative voice of 'the public'. There were extended discussions around sampling issues and the question of representativeness, and participants repeatedly returned to these issues. One person felt that as a pretty fair insight into the values of a wide range of patients and carers emerged from the experience of general practice, GPs on the advisory groups already brought that insight into the public's cares, concerns and priorities into the advisory group process anyway. Was a specific project like the Citizens Council therefore not redundant?

The Council's rejection of the 'fair innings' argument (that younger patients should be privileged over older ones on the grounds that the latter have already had 'a fair innings') had challenged the views of the steering group and indeed of the health economists who worked with NICE. It now caused near disbelief among many of the participants from the appraisals advisory groups. How could the Citizens Council reject so manifestly reasonable a position? Had they heard 'all the hard cases'? They were assured that this was the case and indeed that the leading proponent of the 'fair innings' argument had been among the expert witnesses.

People remained concerned. They discovered from their questioning that there were things not included in the reports that they would have found helpful to know. They wanted more on process. "If we are to be asked to use these views, then how they were arrived at is very important" was how a participant summed up the overall sense of uncertainty in one workshop. Another echoed this:

———

> "If the Citizens Council couldn't agree then that is just as important to know as if they reached a decision, because it shows there is division and conflict around a given issue."

Members of all the advisory groups were agreed on the significance of value judgements as well as technical judgements in their work. The appraisals committees felt that they rejected very few of the technologies they reviewed, "but we do tinker at the margins about who should be given a drug, etc – and that's where the social value judgements come in". In other words, many participants framed value judgements as the tool of last resort, adequate evidence from good research obviating the need for them. Also, where cost-effectiveness required either selectivity or rejection, value judgements became inescapable. One group, noting the lack of weighting in the Council's reports, preferred to wait for the outcome of the survey research on the public's attitudes to QALYs as providing what they felt was a firmer evidence base. Another group, however, was inspired by the whole discussion of social value judgements that arose from the Citizens Council reports into suggesting that 'Guideline considerations' (the document explaining how they 'made the leap' from the evidence to the guideline) could be improved by containing explicit reference to the social value judgements which they had used.

Participants were very aware from their own work of the sometimes disproportionate power of certain witnesses. This made them both empathise with Council members, and be cautious. What was the nature and quality of these 'data' on the public's social values? How were they derived? Were they reliable? What weight was the report going to be given in the Institute's decision-making processes?

At the first workshop, the Chair handled what threatened to become spiralling doubt firmly:

> "It's an experiment; that's why we're evaluating it. So today we want you to engage with how you might use it – it's no use rewriting the method!"

Thus admonished, participants split up into small groups to discuss three set questions. The first asked whether the social value judgements applied in the reports resonated with those applied so far in the work of the advisory committees. The second asked what issues would arise in the incorporation of the Council's value judgements. The

third requested ideas about appropriate processes to demonstrate
that Citizens Council recommendations were being incorporated.
These were all 'how?' questions – they left no space for 'whether?'.

All the groups experienced difficulties with these questions and
the different Council reports, in part because the reports were
internally contradictory. Which parts should they be taking into
account? Which represented the social value judgements of the
Council? Participants in these sessions relied heavily on the
facilitators from the steering group. All the appraisals workshop
groups eventually found that the section in the clinical need report
on 'features of the disease' did resonate with their own discussions
in committee. But the section on 'features of the patient' did not,
because this was more relevant to 'downstream practice'; that is, it
concerned the clinician–patient relationship within which the
technologies appraised by their committees were used, but it did
not enter into discussions at the level of generality at which they
themselves worked in appraisals committees. One group decided
that therefore it might be precisely these 'non-fit features' that they
might need to incorporate more into their discussions:

> "We have to remind ourselves of the patient voice when
> the patient is quiet – and when it [the patient's voice] is
> loud we remind ourselves of all the other patients."

Another group reflected that within their appraisals committee they
did not make reference to features such as age and 'race', even where
they were relevant, because, they felt, of misguided 'political correctness'.
Someone suggested that it might be useful to delegate to a member of
a committee the responsibility for reminding the group of the social
value judgements of the Citizens Council which appeared to be
particularly relevant to a given topic. In one of the guidelines
workshops, however, one participant pointed out that what was
particularly valuable in the Council's reports was precisely this sense
of the whole patient: "whereas in Guidelines we look at specific
conditions; there is a tendency to forget the overall frame which the
Citizens Council reminds us of".

In the plenary sessions, ideas began to emerge from the collation
of the different groups' discussions. Should the Council's reports
be reframed as broad principles for the committees to follow? This
was given a guarded welcome, but overall there was a feeling that
any such principles should not be mandatory. The chair of the
appraisals committees set out two possibilities: a 'hard' approach,

where social value judgements would be specifically referred to in documents, and a 'soft' one, where they might, for example, become part of induction for new members and away-day discussions. The chair of the Institute suggested that the board itself might turn them into guidelines.

The guidelines workshop members became particularly interested in envisaging ways of working collaboratively with the Council. The Council's value lay in its representing 'independent voices' – 'inside but outside'. Could they invite Council members to meet with them and give their views on matters they were wrestling with? One participant found the idea of such a group so inspiring that he said that "this methodology could be useful for the NHS – in our trust we could do with a Citizens Council!". But there were also those who felt that all this was essentially invalid:

> "It is not really finding out the general public's social value judgements, but about setting up a forum where some of the public can discuss these things. It's a very tightly controlled and organised process...."

This was a definition of deliberation as good as any provided by the theorists in Chapter Two. In effect, however, the debate was revealing just how fragile and contestable a deliberative ideal could be when discussed in the context of evidence-based healthcare practice as it was formulated in the Institute.

Taken together, several ideas as to how the outputs of the Citizens Council could be used within the Institute emerged from the four workshops. *Identifying opportunities within the pathways of existing processes* was one. Guidelines groups suggested using the Council's reports as part of the induction of new guideline development groups (these are recruited afresh for each guideline). They also thought that they should "inform the refinement of the remit" – that is, the initial scoping of a new guideline. Appraisals committee members thought that assessment centres' reports to their committees should include them too. Guidelines groups favoured making the value judgements in existing guidelines explicit, and suggested that they could be used in 'Guideline considerations' to explain how they moved from the evidence to the guideline. 'Exception reporting' was another possibility, where a social value judgement could be invoked when a guideline rejected certain evidence. *Mutual agenda setting* was a second proposal. Both appraisals and guidelines groups suggested a role for the Council in deciding which health technologies and which conditions should be examined. Both also wanted to formulate topics for the Citizens Council to discuss. Groups concerned with guidelines were particularly interested in feeding generic questions on which they needed help to the Citizens Council for use with guideline updates. *A principles framework was a third practical idea.* Central guidance on the content of values that had emerged from Council deliberation and on how to use them consistently was suggested.

All the groups expressed the same view that the reports of the Council should be *an information resource* and not be made mandatory. Groups and their members should be aware of them, but be free to disregard them where they felt that their own judgements were more appropriate to the case, giving their reasons. In other words, they should inform the working of the advisory groups, but not dictate it. A decision would be needed as to whether or not an explicit reference to their use or their rejection needed to be made. This 'not mandatory' position paralleled the thinking of many of the commentators on citizens' juries in a local government setting – arguing that while jury findings should be taken into account, the final decision in this case must rest with elected representatives (see Chapter One).

Despite their suspicion regarding the standing and validity of the Council's work, those who attended these impact workshops were positive. They very much regretted not having had the time previously to debate the values surrounding their work, and some commented that they envied the Council its three whole days of discussion on a particular topic. A major impact of the Citizens Council on the Institute was thus to provide the time, the context and the legitimacy for in-house discussion on social value judgements.

As the research team left the scene in the autumn of 2004, the Institute was already involved in further organisational change. The government's review of arm's length bodies had meant absorbing the Health Development Agency, thereby adding public health to NICE's functions and generating considerable internal reorganisation. The Citizens Council continued to meet, from now on in London rather than around the country. Associated with the new public health remit was a new Patient, Carer and Public Involvement Programme (posted on the website on 17 January 2005). The Citizens Council now ranked alongside the Partners Council. A draft consultation document was followed in September 2005 by a paper entitled 'Social value judgements: principles for the development of NICE's guidance'.

Conclusion

Council members acknowledged, as one of their number memorably put it, that they had been on "a knowledge adventure". Members of their host organisation, as this chapter has shown, were also involved in an exploration – devising a new kind of practice and seeking to integrate it with what was more familiar. From an initial position of 'no capture' the Institute moved to a more conversational model of interaction with the Council, understanding rather better what topics were appropriate and how they might be handled. From 'working at one remove' with strong attachment to a 'meta-question', NICE shifted towards topics that linked more to its mainstream activities. Two years on, principles for integrating social value judgements into the work of the Institute were starting to be devised. The Institute was also on the cusp of a fundamental realignment. Citizens Council reports, it was now being argued, should be seen as one resource among others. In reflecting the values of those the NHS served, the Institute's decisions should be influenced by public opinion surveys and focus groups, as well as by the deliberations of its Citizens Council.

Tough questions about this kind of citizen participation had come from several quarters. Was the Council really independent? What was the status of its reports, and how were they to fit with other evidence collected by the Institute? Was it, in the end, worth all the expense? The Institute reflected on and reframed the Citizens Council, revisiting the parameters it had laid down, both in terms of what it perceived a citizen forum would need, and in terms of what it itself needed – as an organisation set up at a particular time and in a particular way.

Throughout this process, the Institute did much to hold to the idea and ideal of citizen deliberation, and it struggled to find ways of fostering its practice. It resisted proposals for example, to reduce the level of resource. And yet, just as the discursive climate in the deliberative assembly itself did not always foster deliberation, that in the host organisation too was not one in which such a notion would find easy acceptance or go unchallenged. Two points can be emphasised here and will start to move us on to the broader themes of Part III. First, there is the pull of what we might call an *individual preferences model*. Consider the way in which the paper on scientific and social value judgements spoke of 'values generally held' by those using the NHS and the move thereafter to engage in opinion polling. This kind of talk and action draws on a notion of the individual as an independent possessor of a bundle of preset opinions or preferences.

It contrasts with the assumptions among deliberation theorists that preferences and choices emerge and develop through the very process of interaction itself. Second, there is the slide towards a *singular reality model*. Participants at one point were faced with different findings from deliberation and from polling. In the end, their response was triangulation. The procedure and indeed the metaphor itself invoke the idea of capturing more dimensions of an essentially single phenomenon by viewing it from different angles. The alternative assumption is that realities are multiple and incommensurate, and that alternative courses of action are not so much uncovered by individual reasoning or by probability sampling, but are constructed through an intersubjective process of deliberation. Deliberators, working well, are thus likely to propose a wider range of relevant factors than had previously been conceived, and novel solutions to a problem can emerge as a result of processes of well-informed, other-regarding, back-and-forth argument that is deliberation. How well does such an argument stand in the light of the case study findings as a whole?

Part III
Implications

EIGHT

Reframing citizen deliberation

NICE's Citizens Council aimed to bring the voices of ordinary citizens into the centre of a key governmental decision-making process in healthcare. Politicians, civil servants, officials and many of the experts associated with the Institute already accepted that in giving advice to ministers about which drugs and treatments should be made available to the NHS, science alone could never be entirely decisive. In each case, there was a value judgement to be made. The Institute's process of stakeholder dialogue already acknowledged this to an important extent; patient groups, clinicians, managers and the pharmaceutical industry had a say. Creating an independent group of citizens bringing the diversity of their own experience alongside this would enable the Institute to keep in touch with the thinking of ordinary people, helping to ensure that the values which underpinned decisions reflected those of health service users as a whole. 'Deliberation' was a procedure which had been gaining in popularity – a process whereby citizens would have access to relevant information, and have the opportunity to discuss and debate and to set out the reasoning that enabled them to come to some conclusions. Coming together for joint reflection in this way would be a different experience for citizens from logging a preference in a survey or via a vote, and the outcome of such informed and shared reflection might well differ significantly from the results of opinion polling. Theorists, furthermore, had advanced some ambitious claims for deliberation – that it had the potential to broaden the range of considerations in a debate, and to generate novel solutions, that it could both enhance citizen capacity and prompt greater legitimacy for decisions in contentious areas.

The Council certainly had an impact both on the citizens and their hosts. Large numbers of citizens came forward to be members. Interviewed after the first four meetings, those selected reported that they had enjoyed the experience – so much so that several were taking steps to find new forms of citizen participation in the future. The Institute, at first unclear, found ways of using the first four reports to develop its thinking and its practice. And yet, a reader looking to these reports for an account of the values of ordinary citizens, set out and reconciled through deliberative reasoning, would emerge disappointed.

We documented considerable unease within the Institute at the first report, and a degree of dissatisfaction and doubt about the process surrounded the reception of the others in the wider Institute community. And in practice, both the clinical need report and the final report on age, far from adding legitimacy, provoked some public challenge from key stakeholder groups. Claims about the potential of deliberation did not seem to have been realised, at least over this first two years.

This was a high profile/high commitment experiment in deliberation. Very considerable resources were set aside to support it, including resources to conduct an ethnographic evaluation. With all the material we were able to amass through close observation of process, what assessments can be made? Should we conclude that the quest for deliberation is a theoreticians' fantasy? Should we be suggesting that decisions with a technical content should after all remain in the hands of the experts, and that members of the public cannot handle complex information? While we lend support to neither of these pessimistic propositions, nor does this study suggest that we should line up in a straightforward way with the optimists who press for an immediate extension of deliberative citizen participation to an ever-widening range of issues and policy topics. The aim of this chapter is to set out and develop an understanding of citizen deliberation which is more in tune with the way in which citizens think, which works with issues of power, and which accommodates 'contextual features' in a nuanced way.

The chapter is in three sections. In the first we briefly summarise key findings from the observation of deliberation in Citizens Council meetings, emphasising just how much of a departure from the ideal model of deliberation these represent. The second section returns to the alternative theoretical framework set out at the end of Chapter Two, moving on from the research questions set out there to guide the empirical work, and taking the analysis of deliberative practice further. The final section moves to the wider context, suggesting how a discursive approach might be of additional value here.

Deliberation in question

Political scientists, as we saw earlier, have expended much effort in exploring deliberation, positioning it as a practice which has the potential to renew democracy by enlarging citizen participation and moving away from adversarial debate to more exploratory and reflective modes of reasoning. Deliberation is understood in this tradition in a hypothetical way – it is about what people would think were they to be exposed to fact and opinion and given an opportunity to discuss with each other and to expand their horizons. Chapter Two teased out from this what we called the deliberative ideal, posing it in stark terms of three moments. These were: an initial statement of positions, the hearing of evidence and argumentation, and the production of other-regarding reasoning, aimed at finding a position capable of accommodating difference. A great deal of effort, as that chapter indicated, has gone into identifying and debating the salience of factors which might limit the realisation of this understanding of deliberation.

There is no doubt that the deliberative assembly studied here operated in ways that were distant from the deliberative ideal in the sense outlined. The first meeting generated a particularly confused and confusing result. Simple quantitative measures of the volume of focused questions and deliberative exchanges demonstrated that these were rarities. Close analytical attention to the transcripts showed a highly unsatisfactory result; the design of the key review sessions seemed to freeze out deliberation as participants struggled to recall previous information and comment, without the benefit of a pool of deliberative reasoning on which to draw. While quantitative measures showed an improvement in later meetings, the amount of deliberation continued to be minimal and was often on topics to the side of the main theme of the event.

Questioning of witnesses varied. A particularly impenetrable topic set for the first meeting, together with a large number of witnesses, exacerbated problems. Although the proportion of focused questions was to rise markedly in later meetings, topics framed largely within the discursive world of the host organisation continued to cause difficulty. One factor that made a difference, we were able to show, was a witness who was clearly positioned for or against an issue, and who energetically advocated a particular line. A highly positioned witness, we argued, stimulates the audience to interact and to work out their own response.

Emotional investment not only from witnesses but also among the citizens themselves visibly oiled the wheels of deliberation. Willingness to deliberate increased, for example, when citizens were asked to engage in role-play and were assigned a particular position to argue. They entered imaginatively into this and developed an investment in the outcome. Role-plays helped to identify just what the different positions might be and what thinking underpinned them. In principle, facilitation could work towards the same result, but here there was a dilemma.

Facilitating to encourage inclusion, and to ensure that all who wished to speak had an opportunity to do so, served to cut deliberation short. It identified topics and positions but moved between them without providing space to explore associated reasoning. Techniques introduced in later meetings – such as working in pairs then moving to a small and a larger group, or producing and revisiting individual written responses – brought out more articulation of reasoning and encouraged and allowed changes of mind.

There were fragments of deliberation in the sense of reflective debate among diverse group members influenced by available information. These stayed vividly in the minds of some Council members as personally enriching and enlarging experiences. Interviewed later, one for example gave an instance from the first meeting where she had come to see the value of a hospital prayer room. In another interview, there was a tantalising glimpse of a challenge to the 'fair innings' argument for prioritising health services on age grounds – identifying it as a specifically middle-class standpoint. It is discouraging for advocates of deliberation, however, that such points found clearest expression not in the assembly itself but, later, in individual interviews. More encouraging perhaps, was the testimony in final interviews that people had enjoyed hearing new viewpoints, teasing out what prompted them, and reflecting on the reasoning involved. Some Council members, interestingly, saw fit in the induction for new members to warn them that they would change their minds several times during the event and 'this is OK'. As one put it, "we don't have to agree, but you have to know what you think".

All four of the areas of critique that we identified from the deliberation literature were pertinent in this case study and the material offers strong support for their relevance. On the theme of *power, pluralism and oppression*, our findings do much to confirm the concerns of the critics. The analysis of the 'clapping incident' in Chapter Six provides a vivid example of the dilemmas produced by hegemonic discourses around political correctness and majoritarian views, and the difficulty both of mounting an oppositional standpoint in the Council itself and of persuading the group that ground rules need to be set in order for this to occur. On deliberation theory's prohibition of *arguing from interests*, and instead producing 'justifications that can be acknowledged by all', several observations can be made. For one thing, there was little at any point in the proceedings that could be seen as the advancement of an interest by Council members. Far from always bringing established positions or interests to the debate, these 'unhyphenated citizens' struggled to find a position from which to speak. And without clear access to established positions, deliberation theory's imagined rhetorical device of other-regarding exchanges become difficult to articulate. It was notable, too, that participants, early on at least, were strongly motivated towards producing a consensus and worried about how any conflicting views could be reconciled. Asserting a differential identity and the experience that flowed from it seemed altogether too risky a business. Questions of *knowledge, expertise and experience* also proved challenging. Efforts to inform through formal witness presentations were rarely successful and the expertise space for citizens *qua* citizens, we concluded in Chapter Six, was fragile and contested – including by citizens themselves. Finally, there is the question of *sanitised debate* and messy practice. Not surprisingly, perhaps, the opportunity to observe deliberation at such close quarters moved us firmly into the 'messy' camp. Practical deliberation, as more and more of the theorists now acknowledge, does not fit the neat, staged categories of moments of information receipt, and information digesting, followed by other-regarding exchanges.

One possible interpretation of all this would be to suggest that this Citizens Council was a special case, not to be equated with the more 'successful' citizens' jury initiatives. Compared, for example, with the citizens' jury initiatives which have attracted strongly positive commentaries (see Chapter Two), it created a larger and more unwieldy group; the questions were not concrete and immediate, but abstract and discursively unfamiliar. There is something to be said for this special case argument. Certainly it seemed that as the question became more concrete, so the ease with which citizens were able to engage increased. But the struggle with the question also helped to reveal the unrealistic assumptions of a model of deliberation not firmly grounded in everyday reasoning and social interaction. This we pursue in the following sections.

A related set of objections might focus on the Council as altogether too much of a creature of the host organisation. Compared with many one-off citizens' juries, the Council was in a complex and more enduring relationship with its host organisation, and as such more open to the possibility, of which the Institute was only too aware, of manipulation and capture. Ironically perhaps, the very appreciation of this danger, and the intent strongly expressed at the outset not to capture the citizens, exacerbated matters, since the Council was left in the dark about how the questions it was asked related to the powers and responsibilities of NICE. It remained the case, however, that the Institute set the questions; the Institute made the decisions about the witnesses, it employed the facilitators, and its steering group was involved at every point in the decisions about format and design. In formal terms, too, the Council was advisory – it was the board of the Institute that received reports and decided on any action.

A third potential line of interpretation might be to stress 'design faults'. In our final report on the evaluation, we were able to identify some of the factors that encouraged deliberation. These were much as others have already noted, setting a very clear question, using a variety and array of imaginative techniques and 'games' to explore implications and allocating substantial resources to facilitation, although, as we have observed, inclusive facilitation can have a contradictory character, and requires more attention (Davies et al, 2005). The argument of this chapter, however, is that more needs to be done than the mere identification of 'what works' if we are to advance understanding and devise citizen-friendly practices. Deliberation, as presently construed, is too far from the everyday, and as such it makes unrealistic assumptions. There is a need "to work with the grain of how citizens behave", recognising that "to work against the grain is to reproduce the passive citizen" (Prior et al, 1995: 88). There is also a need to find a means of unpicking the context of a deliberative initiative, examining the ways in which it both affects and is affected by the practice of deliberation, and integrating this also into novel forms of theorising.

Practice, discourse and the deliberative ideal

What happens when we view the findings of this book not through the lens of conventional political science argumentation on deliberation, but through the lens of social practice? Practice theory offers the notion that the coordination of activities brings new situations into being. People both reproduce the familiar and continually customise their actions *in situ*, in a process of mutual engagement and sense making. Regularities and patterning emerge in the creation of a community of practice. The exchanges that occur are historically situated, in the sense that participants call on culturally available discursive resources to position themselves, and to give meaning to what is occurring. The nature of these resources, and the commitments and assumptions built into them, need critical and deconstructive examination. Discourse theory, we argued in Chapter Two, has the capacity to do this, putting flesh on an abstract notion of practice, and showing how subject positions, including, crucially, the subject position of the citizen, are constituted and reconstituted. Our initial research questions reflected this. They were to do with the forms of discursive practice that develop in a deliberative assembly, the elements that come to form a community of practice, and how power plays out in live contexts. What new insights into the deliberative process can be gleaned from this?

There are several ways in which use of a practice approach provides an alternative to the deliberation ideal, offering contrasting assumptions and ones more deeply grounded in the actuality of everyday discourse. Three of these will be discussed in turn below with reference to the findings we have already presented. First, there is the question of *what citizens bring* into a deliberative arena. This relates to values and commitments, the thorny issue for the deliberation theory of 'interests', and also to the important matter of discursive styles. Second, through the unfolding dynamic of interaction there is *the emergence of a community of practice*. We will argue that this is by no means something that can be pre-designed and given to a deliberative assembly, although what is pre-designed is part of the unfolding mix. Including one final excerpt from the corpus of data, we also argue that a collaborative form of interaction, rather than the much discussed deliberative ideal, better meets the hopes that have been invested in visions of deliberation. Thirdly and most crucially, there is the way in which practice theory expresses and analyses *power*.

What do citizens bring?

Citizens Council members had put themselves forward for this experiment in citizen participation for a variety of reasons. Some told us that they had a sense of public duty and wanted to give something back; others had responded directly to the cue in the advertisement about making improvements in the NHS. Several felt that this would be an opportunity for personal development – it would stretch them and 'exercise the brain' to try something new. For all Council members, as Chapter Six noted, deliberation became pre-eminently a practical problem. What was the appropriate way to comport oneself in this unfamiliar situation? There was some sense of end goals (a report and recommendations) and some structures were in place (witness sessions, plenaries etc), but considerable ambiguity remained about what might be seen as 'doing a good job'.

Members of the Council were not entirely in the dark in all this, however, and practice theory gives a basis for analysing the discursive resources that they bring. Bakhtinian theory (see Morson and Emerson,

1990) suggests that these resources will consist of a heteroglossia of genres from everyday practices and life worlds. Any new discursive situation thus becomes constructed out of the patchwork of discursive styles available to each participant, and the way in which these are selected *in situ* and in response to the utterances of others. The mix-on-the-day is never entirely predictable. Each emerging practice, furthermore, carries with it the history of its past use – its contexts, its evaluative and ethical tones, its subject positions, its points of view, its ideological dilemmas, its accents and intonations – the very flavours of the whole way of life in which it has been primarily previously used (cf Maybin, 2001). We saw the complexity of these features at work, for example, in the different styles that citizens came to employ, as 'researcher', 'interrogator' and 'chair'. We saw it at another level, in the way that norms of politeness and of political correctness were invoked and shared by a majority, but, significantly, not by all present. Thus, although the Citizens Council, meeting for the first time, had zero history in itself, the mix of discursive practices which came to constitute it trail behind them convoluted histories which will not necessarily achieve deliberation theory's goal of free and equal exchange. Chapter Six demonstrated that a discursive analysis offers the possibility of understanding the ways in which hegemonic discourses become inserted into the practices of a deliberative arena through the actions of participants. A forum intended as democratic, in this way can become undemocratic. In short, a deliberative event can never be a fresh discursive start or a bubble independent of other contexts. New theorising, and new deliberative initiatives, must acknowledge and work with what people bring.

It is not that deliberation theorists ignore what is brought in to the deliberative arena; it is rather that the way in which they characterise it needs to be called into question. Thus, their call for the statement and transformation of positions in the course of a meeting is built on a well-established tradition in western thought that sees an attitude or an opinion as an internal state of mind, and an individual possession – a fixed and enduring personal trait, portable and thus importable into a deliberation. This assumes that when the moment comes for expressing views, individuals will simply scrutinise the internal mental states that they have brought and will report on them. Studies in discursive psychology (Potter and Wetherell, 1987; Edwards and Potter, 1992) have done much to contest this individualistic and cognitivist approach to public opinion. A corpus of work by Michael Billig on rhetoric, arguing and thinking makes this particularly plain (Billig, 1987, 1991; Billig et al, 1988). He explains:

> Rarely, if ever, is the giving of an opinion merely a spontaneous report of an internal state. If somebody says 'I feel that capital punishment is wrong' they are unlikely to be making a claim to be reporting a particular internal state of feeling, which only occurs when the topic of capital punishment arises and which is attached to no other topic. Their utterance is likely to be part of a conversation and its meaning should be analysed in terms of the conversational context.... A statement in favour of capital punishment is not merely a report about the speaker's self-positioning on the issue. Nor is it merely a statement about what the speaker supports. It is also a positioning against counter positions.... In this sense, the statement of an opinion often indicates a readiness to argue on a matter of controversy. (Billig, 2001: 214)

Extracts 9 and 18 in earlier chapters of this study provide illustration of this point, underlining that, in the context of deliberation, people's opinions, evaluative statements and preferences are likely to be tentative, enmeshed in dialogue, and variable over time and context. The significance of work in this discursive vein is to demonstrate that in practice, argumentation unfolds moment by moment, with each utterance designed to fit the previous pattern of utterances. Opinion giving is thus not the solipsistic revelation of a consistent and logical pattern of thoughts, coherently pre-ordered in individual minds. Indeed, because utterances are designed to fit the back and forth of conversational flow, it is often not meaningful to ask who 'owns' a particular thought and it is certainly not appropriate to assume that that thought is a something that an individual somehow 'brings' into the room. We have repeatedly seen in the chapters of Part II the tensions that can be produced for those designing deliberation if they make the assumption, consistent with much deliberation theory to date, that there are pre-established preferences and values and that these can be uncovered, given the right mix of facilitation exercises and techniques.

An emerging community of practice

Turning from what people bring to how they engage in social interaction, deliberation theory, as we saw in Chapter Two, has made important moves in recent years away from 'sanitised' debate and other-regarding exchanges, towards a more encompassing notion of what is actually likely to take place in the deliberative arena, accepting, for example, rhetoric, narrative and humour. The ethnographic data bear this out, and a discourse analytic approach, paying attention to how a community of practice gets established, adds both depth and complexity to this position. In the first meeting, exacerbated by the complexity of the question being asked, participants were uneasy and subdued in their casting about for cues as to how to question witnesses, and how to engage with each other in addressing the question. Already by the second meeting, however, there was more familiarity and ease and signs, if not of an entirely settled view of 'how we do things', then at least of a settling view. Different styles and genres were offered in this emerging community of practice; they were filtered through assessments of each other (in what was a more diverse group than almost any had previously experienced), through tentative understandings of what was proper in a public venue that was still unfamiliar to many, and through pleasure, for example, in the rhetorical devices of debate, recognised as familiar from the mass media. Not all forms of interaction were equally valued, however. We have given attention to the uncertain place of narrative, stories of personal experience and anecdote and to the squeezing out of minority discourses – this latter a particularly worrying result to which we return below.

Moments of sustained and reflective exchange between two or more participants occurred as summarised earlier in this chapter when participants were emotionally engaged and when witnesses, for example, were clearly positioned. But there is more to say about the deliberative character of this emerging community of practice. The final extract set out below stems from a small group session in the third meeting. Here several members of the Council muse over the relevance, if any, of a person's social role to their access to health treatment. The floor is shared between several speakers, all contributing different threads to a common topic. The emotional mood or tone is of collective and cooperative puzzling to find an answer. The interaction here has a number of discursive features. 'Duetting' often occurs, or the finishing of each other's utterances or chains of thought. Speakers often end on a question that then draws an answer from another speaker, a clarification, or a new example from a previous speaker. The discussion is good-humoured, there is a cumulative progression as the group works through possible positions and, in this example, the nature of the dilemma clearly emerges.

Extract 23

Cindy: "I mean if you don't look at it maybe you would miss out. It's like what would, say age should be an informing factor, not a determining one. Social role, you know ..."

Graham: "Mmm ..."

Cindy: "Social role, you know, could be a very, very minor part that you take on board but it ..."

Joan: "Should be a part of it."

Cindy: "Yeah ..."

Alan: "Or you can end the other way where he's laid on the ... operating, a person on the operating table and the surgeon just going through his CV first to see if he's working [laughter]. [multiple voices] That's how the extremes start by one person changing one rule. That's how the extremes start."

Joan: "So you're saying a social role is ... the fact that he's working maybe the social role could be someone who doesn't work but actually has a great role within a lot of voluntary organisations." [multiple voices]

Cindy: "Say the guy was a bus driver, yes. And he comes into A&E and he collapses, and somebody looks at his wallet and finds out he's a bus driver. Right, now they're going to phone up the bus company and say 'look I'm really sorry this guy's been in an accident'."

James: "... and the bus is going to be metered ..."

Cindy: "Can't be at work. So in that sense his social role is important." [background noise]

Graham: "Yeah, but we're on about his social role determining whether he gets treatment or not?"

> Facilitator: [inaudible]
>
> Nigel: "How can you decide that, that?"
>
> Anoop: "But we could look at the bigger picture, we wouldn't just look at, I assume, just that ,would we?"
>
> Graham: "I just can't see social role being any other than being discriminatory."
>
> Nigel: "How could you decide? How could you decide?"
>
> Shefique: "It's going to discriminate affect everyone doesn't it?"
>
> Nigel: "That bus driver is more important than the voluntary worker, than the MP, than the mother with the children?"
>
> Cindy: "Yeah."
>
> Nigel: "How can you, how can you make that division?"
>
> Alan: "That [inaudible] ..."
>
> Nigel: "And make a list and or table and give points depending on that. You couldn't, no."

Of the varied discursive practices demonstrated in the Council meetings, exchanges like this come closest to what theorists and advocates mean by deliberation. Crucially, however, this exchange does not entail positions being taken by individuals and defended through other-regarding exchanges. Instead it is a more collaborative form, involving multiple participants in a process of jointly reflective and open-ended discussion. An examination of all of the back–and–forth exchanges included in our basic quantitative measure of deliberation revealed that, while some were adversarial in nature (in the set piece role-plays, for example, and in relation to particular witnesses), it was more common for these exchanges to take this collaborative form. This collaborative and exploratory style was also evident in some of the active engagements with witnesses as well as in those between Council members themselves.

It is not, then, merely that deliberative theory needs to consider how humour, rhetoric and anecdote can be added to the deliberative process. It is rather that the fundamentals of deliberation itself need rethinking, in order to move beyond simplistic procedural models based on ideals of good argument to a more nuanced, encompassing understanding of the actuality of interaction between citizens. What, then, of the third theme we have identified?

Question of power

Power has been a perennial theme in deliberation theory. The common denominator in definitions of deliberation to date is that it is interaction occurring without coercion, strategising or manipulation. For deliberation to work, the theorists seem to say, power must be eliminated. Power here is conceptualised as force exercised directly by one participant over another. Theorists speculate how far it can be neutralised, for example, by the public character of the event, or by ground rules emphasising the task as a quest for the common good. The present analytical frame rejects such a starting point, seeking to show that the power relations circulating around a deliberative assembly have little to do with direct coercion and rarely involve the strategic manipulation of others. This form of analysis, influenced by Foucauldian scholars, emphasises not only the controlling but also the constructing character of power. We have shown how patterns of social advantage and disadvantage embedded in the discursive practices brought to the Council, plus the forms of speaking which are validated by powerful others, give content and flavour to the event. We have shown, too, how widely shared norms of politeness, for example, and of equal-as-identical treatment can effectively preclude the emergence of oppositional discourses. Power in this sense is thus conveyed through what is taken for granted, what seems normal and natural; its effects are subtle and emergent – often obvious only with hindsight.

The 'clapping incident' (Chapter Six) provided one of the clearest examples of the way in which power comes to reproduce hegemonic discourse. The moment when those from the host organisation brought citizens deep into the debate process on one particular drug appraisal – that of Cox II inhibitors for treatment of pain in arthritis – was perhaps another (Chapter Five). Council members were emotionally and cognitively engaged; the discussion sessions facilitated the emergence of reasoning that they could share, and the result echoed that of the appraisal committee itself. What are we to make of such a conclusion? Did this moment of practice serve to create an expertise space from which citizens could speak as citizens, or did it bring citizens as 'good pupils' into an appreciation of the expertise space of NICE itself, to produce an echo of the outcomes achieved there?

This brings us back once again to the key question of the circumstances under which oppositional ideas and arguments emerge and can be sustained. The need for such alternative ideas, counter-argument and oppositional discourses is fundamental to the ideal of deliberation as producing novel and inclusive possibilities (Dryzek, 2000a). We saw in Chapter Six that citizens' ideas about appropriate forms of public debate served to sap their confidence that their life world narratives could be good enough for this arena. Could it be that the deliberative ideal, grounded as it is in the work of Habermas and his notion of an ideal speech situation, undermines rather than supports citizen efforts? Theorist Jessica Kulynych suggests that this is so:

> The model of an ideal speech situation establishes a norm of rational interaction that is defined by the very types of interaction that it excludes.... Defining an ideal speech inevitably entails defining unacceptable speech ... speech evocative of identity, culture or emotion has no necessary place in the ideal speech situation....Therefore, a definition of citizenship based on participation in an ideal form of interaction can easily become a tool for the exclusion of deviant communicators from the category of citizens. (1997: 324-5; cf Young, 1996)

What is needed, she argues, is a Habermas more sensitive to Foucault, an argument, that is, that can encompass performative power and the micro-politics of resistance. The outcome of her closely argued consideration of Foucault on power and resistance is not a call for rational dialogue, but for the enactment of a drama, or the creative theatre of a political demonstration, that serves to expose, reveal and literally 'demonstrate' oppression and subjection. By such imaginative and creative means, "that which cannot be argued for finds expression" (Kulynych, 1997: 334). There was some use of such techniques in the Citizens Council. They have been deployed more extensively in some of the more radical citizens' jury models, in the nano-jury, for example (see Chapter One). Theatre may not be the whole of the answer to deliberation, but these theoretical arguments bring us back once again to the limits of procedural approaches to deliberation. They misunderstand the significance of identity and emotional engagement to the flow of power. They fail to sustain the very democratic exchanges they seek to instate. A Habermasian, procedural account is never going to be sufficient as a model for deliberation and a yardstick for its measurement.

In sum: in the detailed case study analysis of this book, we have shown that inequalities and social divisions enter with citizens in the very discursive resources they invoke. We have suggested that deliberation theory has sought to instate its particular vision of practice: (a) without understanding the significance and complexity of the heteroglossic practices which people will bring into a new arena; (b) without confronting and allowing a theoretical place for ways in which the old, the new and the different will intertwine; (c) without appreciating the possibilities and limits of dialogue as generative of positions and preferences, as a source of value clarification and also, perhaps, of interest formation; and (d) without engaging with the subtlety and complexity of the power relations that circulate in the discursive practices in use. We have also indicated not just that the deliberative ideal fails to accommodate the actuality of social practice, but, as Kulynych suggests, that it can work against the very generative dialogue it seeks to instate. The deliberative ideal as *outcome* (expanded notions of the possible, collaborative dialogue about the preferable) is one thing; but the deliberative ideal as *procedure*, in the shape of a quest to reproduce the ideal speech situation, is in question.

And yet the analysis cannot end here. Commentators hostile to deliberation frequently leave aside the specificities of practice within a deliberative arena to argue that ultimately it is institutional and organisational forms that keep existing power relations intact, and limit the possibilities for citizens to engage. An adequate theory of citizen participation thus needs to deal with these more meso- and macro-considerations. How important is the overall context of participatory initiatives and the organisational arrangements and specific design of a deliberative assembly? What can an ethnographic study and an approach from discourse and social practice offer here?

Constructing context and constraint

While deliberation theory has focused in the main on prescriptions for the conduct of deliberation, academics have also been to the fore in creating and running practical examples of deliberation. A body of evaluative commentary has grown up offering practical recommendations for how to design and run events, drawing from this experience (see Chapter Two). Sceptics, however, as we have seen, argue that forms of citizen participation and involvement are always open to manipulation by elites, that deliberative initiatives either do not have the degree of structural autonomy and control that will allow them to come up with novel ideas, or that, if this is the case, there is almost never any guarantee that recommendations will be implemented.

It is certainly clear that there are many aspects of design and implementation at the meso-level that have the potential to contain, control and limit a deliberative event. Stirling (2005) offers a particularly long list of what he calls 'contingencies', covering the dynamics of the deliberation itself but also ranging, for example, from the nature of the relationship with sponsors and the engagement of stakeholders to the boundaries of the remit, the management of information and so on (see Chapter Two). A feature of the research on which this book is based, however, was that it included not just a detailed ethnography of deliberative interactions, but also an analysis of the context in which that deliberation took place. Utilising concepts from discourse analysis and from practice theory has enabled us to frame 'the context' (or 'contingencies') not as an entirely pre-given and settled set of constraints, but, to an important extent, as actively constructed and reconstructed by key players. These constructions and reconstructions occur in the light of participants' struggles to see possibilities and analyse events – linking all this to the imagined responses of key stakeholders. How did this work?

Chapter One sought to place initiatives in citizen participation within the specific discursive framework of contemporary politics in the UK, showing their entanglement with the New Labour project of rebuilding public confidence, and with intellectual ideas about a new kind of politics, at once more generative of new solutions and more capable of providing legitimation and integration for an increasingly diverse citizenship. It demonstrated the fragility of efforts to establish new kinds of participation in the questioning culture that surrounds today's political interventions, and the potential for disillusion. The climate that has seen the rise and rise of citizen participation, we intimated, is by no means straightforwardly supportive of it. The 'macro-context' in this form of analysis turns out to be a complex and contradictory mix of cultural ideas, political projects and techniques – a mix in which academic ideas about deliberation and the deliberative ideal have themselves become a resource.

Such an assemblage will give citizen participation a particular flavour and meaning in its passage through institutions and organisations. Thus we went on to examine how a new-style regulatory institution, itself fashioned and given legitimacy in important part through the New Labour project, and charged with creating a stakeholder consensus around decisions on healthcare, struggled to make sense of an imperative to add a form of direct citizen participation to its still fairly newly established activities. In putting flesh on the idea of a Citizens Council, NICE filtered its thinking through a series of narratives about the Institute itself, as it constructed its distinctive task and its ways of working in face of an array of often sceptical stakeholders. Members of the Institute also drew from knowledge of citizens' juries, knowledge that was located both among its own staff and in the Department of Health. But they modified the citizens' jury idea substantially. Some will argue that these modifications effectively neutered the Council and corralled the citizens' voices through positioning the Council as an advisory body discussing nebulous values rather than concrete problems. Others will point out that the modifications were pragmatically and positively driven by the need to accommodate the Council to already established stakeholder dialogue. Techniques and practices guiding the actual Council itself were largely settled before the facilitation team was recruited. But these were revisited both in the course of the meetings themselves by the facilitation team, and in subsequent steering group meetings by members of the host organisation in discussion with the facilitators. As we later saw, this resulted in substantial changes to the design and timetable of sessions.

This form of analysis rests heavily on the discursive turn in organisation theory and on the argument that "phenomena such as 'the organisation' ... do not have a straightforward and unproblematic existence independent of our discursively-shaped understandings" (Chia, 2000: 513). Such an approach rejects 'the organisation' and its 'environment' as ontological fixtures, referring instead to 'organising' as a process infused with power, and as constantly becoming. Formally constituted organisations are thus full of "subtle micro-changes that sustain and, at the same time, potentially corrode stability" (Tsoukas and Chia, 2002: 568; cf Weick, 1979). From this perspective, actors in organisations, as elsewhere in social life, must be conceived of:

> ... as webs of beliefs and habits of action that keep reweaving (and thus altering) as they try coherently to

accommodate new experiences, which come from new
interactions over time. (Tsoukas and Chia, 2002: 575)

Drawing from earlier, classic writing in this vein, we began Chapter
Three with Karl Weick's (1979) concept of sense making, and with
his memorable phrase about how individuals 'unrandomise' variables,
in the process creating order and creating constraints. It follows from
this that it is only through close ethnographic observation, tracking
the flows of power, attending to practitioner accounts and the shifting,
reflexive understandings that these represent, that we can understand
settings and organisations and the way that innovations, including the
Citizens Council initiative, will be, not shaped once and for all, but
constituted and reconstituted within them.

All this is not necessarily to commit to a position that organisations
are 'all talk' and can be reinvented at whim, any more than it is to say
that they are all imperatively controlled action and contingency. Reed
(2004), for example, argues that at any point in time actors will be
faced with what he calls "pre-existing authoritative and allocative orders
generated by earlier phases of institution-building". Thus:

> Institutional fields and organisational forms will be shaped
> and reshaped as a result of the complex dialectical interplay
> between pre-existing structural constraints and the
> combined collective efforts of corporate agents to engage
> in new modes of discursive practice that will inevitably
> change them, to some degree or another. (Reed, 2004:
> 416)

One does not necessarily have to subscribe to Reed's critical realist
argument to acknowledge the influence of prior discursive settlements
and sedimented practices from the past. What counts as 'the past' is
always, of course, open to redefinition in the present. But Reed is
right to direct attention to ways in which past practice acts to constrain
present possibilities.

Bakhtinian theory offers a rather different perspective in its
invitation to see the world in terms of what are termed 'centripetal'
and 'centrifugal' forces (cf Morson and Emerson, 1990: 30). In most
cultural situations, the argument goes, one can distinguish forces
for official order (centripetal) and forces that disrupt this order
(centrifugal). Centripetal forces attempt to create a communicative
totality with defined and seemingly fixed features, to systematise
and prescribe, and to identify and enforce 'proper ways of talking'

and proper modes of conduct and interaction which signify, produce and reproduce social institutions. Centrifugal forces at the same time disorganise systems, create exceptions and resist attempts at order. Theorisations such as these are important in resisting those traditions that give firm ontological status to social structures that constrain and in opening up alternative possibilities for understanding how 'constraints' and 'contexts' come to have a character that is both to some extent fixed, yet ultimately also unfixable.

There are further illustrations of these points, if one turns from the policy context in which the Citizens Council was initiated, to its continuing development. The rhythms and practices of the more established communities of practice that make up the Institute created different moments when the significance of the Citizens Council and the relevance of citizen participation to the work of the Institute were debated. We examined three. These were: the point where the steering group considered what there was to learn from the first meeting of the Citizens Council; the point where the Partners Council and then the board rehearsed positions about the value of the Council; and the point, rather later, when internal workshops were set up to tease out just how the output of the Council could be used, and what the next steps should be in bringing a citizen voice and citizen participation into the Institute. These, we argued in Chapter Seven, represented times of discursive challenge, of reframing and repair. On each occasion, internal accounts of what the Council was and how it worked were embellished; each time they crystallised a little more through the processes of rebuttal.

We were able to dwell in particular depth on the exchanges that occurred in the four in-house workshops, set up to consider how to use the output of the Citizens Council. Here again the contestable nature of a deliberative initiative emerged. Questions were repeatedly put concerning how representative the Council was, how well informed its members had become and how robust the process was as compared, for example, with opinion polling. Unlike at the micro-level of the meetings themselves, participants here were not all necessarily invested in making deliberation work. Indeed, the reverse could be the case – the Citizens Council held the potential to disrupt the stakeholder negotiation that was the established appraisal process in the Institute and the advisory forum that was its Partners Council.

Prominent among the discursive moves in the context of the

workshops was the appeal to the evidential standards of science that permeated the practice of the Institute. Assembled together for the workshops were social actors familiar with scientific reasoning and strongly committed to the value of critically appraising evidence. Their 'dominant language game' (Barge, 1994, 2002) had its roots in rationality and logic – in "a set of ordered statements that includes claims, data, warrants, backing, qualifiers, and reservations" (Meyers and Brashers, 2002: 142). In such a context, it could seem impossible that credence could be given to a small group, not satisfactorily representative in any statistical sense, and whose command of the relevant information base could perhaps be questioned. And indeed, challenges of this sort proliferated. But 'context', we have just argued, is multilayered and complex; it is actively interpreted and resisted. Power is uneven. A dominant discursive frame does not always produce winning arguments. The close analysis that we were able to provide showed how the force of science or 'evidence-based' discourse clashed with 'values' discourse and in this case, also, with institutional power. There was an acknowledgement that value judgements entered the appraisal process and that science alone could never be entirely decisive. Practical experience of the limits of scientific reasoning in the daily practice of producing appraisals of drugs and other interventions led some participants at least to call for additional uses of the Citizens Council, bringing its members, for example, more directly into individual appraisals. In the second place, there was the matter of the Council as an initiative that had its origins and legitimation in government health policy. The chair firmly warned critics that "you can't redesign the method".

The Citizens Council emerged from these and further debates framed in a new way. It was to continue with a somewhat reduced budget. It was portrayed as having influenced the in-house production of a paper on dealing with value judgements that then went out for wider consultation. Particularly significantly, it was now positioned as one of several ways in which the Institute was going to be in touch with broader public opinion. There were some in the workshop debates who understood that the point of deliberation was to explore and develop an opinion through exchanges with diverse others – something necessarily different from what might be gathered through opinion polling. There were others, however, who advocated polling as a self-evident means, through triangulation, of checking the validity of the recommendations made. The different discourses in play had given rise to a set of accommodations that arguably had diluted the concept of the Council as a deliberative assembly.

The approach that we are developing here for understanding the meso-, organisational context bears, too, on the vexed question that policy makers and policy analysts often refer to as the 'implementation gap'. It is one thing to appreciate that the conditions for 'perfect implementation' of any policy initiative will never be met (Hogwood and Gunn, 1984). It is another to shift the theoretical focus decisively away from the somewhat mechanical notion of 'implementation', towards an examination of the discourses and the flows of power that construct and reconstruct policy all the way from the very earliest stages through to anticipated and unanticipated change on the ground. One way forward for future research suggested by this study is perhaps to seek to identify sites of discursive engagement in the policy community at meso- and macro-level, and to concentrate ethnographic work in these settings. We did not have access, for example, to the in-house discussion that preceded meetings of the board and the Partners Council. Nor were we able to glean any direct observation data on the Institute's relations with the Department of Health – a key site of interaction given the 'intermediary' position in which the Institute as a regulatory body was placed (Davies, forthcoming). Calls for more interpretive studies in the public policy field head in such a direction (Bevir and Rhodes, 2003; Bevir, 2004).

To summarise: what we are suggesting in this section is not an analysis that works rigidly to identify macro- and meso-level structural relationships and sees these as setting firm limits on micro-level activity, but instead an analysis in which macro-level discourses infuse and inform understanding of the possibilities for social action at different levels. Scientific procedure and its associated quest for rational reasoning, we have argued, made multiple appearances (including, of course, within the Citizens Council), but it did not always and exclusively secure the winning argument. Active reworkings and reweavings of constraints occurred, as these were narrated and re-narrated in the course of daily organisational life. The consequences had some decisive effects on what citizens could do and on the still unfolding, still contested relations of power. Through ethnographic and discursively inflected analysis, in short, we have sought to produce a more nuanced understanding of how discourses and institutions work at the meso- and macro-levels, and to understand in more depth the key point that *deliberative assemblies operate in a wider climate that gives a decidedly mixed endorsement to the practice they seek to instate.*

Conclusion

This chapter has sought to identify new directions for studies of citizen participation – directions released from the orthodoxies of deliberation theory on the one hand, and from notions of structures of constraint and pre-given power relations on the other. Deliberation theory emerges from this ethnographic enquiry as *too cerebral, too homogenising and too universalising in its ambition*. It leads too easily, for example, towards a heavy reliance on information-packed witness presentations. It does not have strategies that are strong enough to risk, encourage and respect difference and conflicts of interest among citizens. Citizens Council members testified that moments of expanded consciousness and mind changing did occur – but differential reasoning and the logics of contrasting value positions failed to emerge with the kind of clarity that could pose in new ways the dilemmas that their host organisation faced, let alone point to directions for their potential resolution. An appropriate expertise space for citizens never fully emerged. Furthermore, as this book has repeatedly shown, deliberation always takes place in a context. Consistent with the social practice theorising that underpinned the observation of the Council in action, we have provided an analysis of 'context' not as a set of fixed constraints, but as a set of interlinked discursive frames. This meant seeing this instance of participation as part of a contradictory New Labour project with its hopes and its moments of disillusion, and tracking through how the idea of the Citizens Council took shape, filtered through successive moments of sense making in NICE. What emerged was the fragility of the idea of citizen participation in the face of more hegemonic discourses.

But if the import of the study as explored in this chapter is to point an academic audience towards the greater use of social practice theory and of discourse analysis, what messages does it convey to an audience concerned with questions of policy and politics? Is there a place at all for citizens at the centre, engaging in deliberation as part of a project of democratic renewal? If there is, how can it be developed to fullest effect?

NINE

New directions for
policy and practice

> What we need, then, are 'real utopias': utopian ideals that
> are grounded in the real potentials of humanity, utopian
> destinations that have pragmatically accessible waystations,
> utopian designs of institutions that can inform our practical
> tasks of muddling through in a world of imperfect
> conditions for social change. (Olin Wright, 2003: vii)

How feasible is it, we asked at the outset of this book, to call on
ordinary people to come forward and take part in decision making,
not just locally but in relation to the institutions of central government?
Is there a viable space for participating citizens at the centre of the
institutions of a democratic state? Visions of politics with places for
citizens – both locally and at the centre – have loomed ever larger in
recent years. Chapter One charted the rise and rise of citizen
participation initiatives in Britain, the growing quest, through citizens'
juries, people's panels and more, to find ways of engaging not just the
organised stakeholders or those directly affected by the outcome of an
issue in political debate, but of creating opportunities to inform those
without an immediate personal interest in the outcome, and to observe
how they might approach an issue, and what arguments might be
persuasive in their ears. Would what we have called 'unhyphenated
citizens' – those without a pressing interest as residents in an area, for
example, or as users of a service – come forward at all? Could they
and would they engage in deliberation? And if these questions could
be answered satisfactorily, what would this mean for existing lines of
authority and relations of political accountability? Just where does
democratic deliberation fit in 21st-century forms of democracy?

The prominent group of scholars in the US who came together
under the banner of the 'Real Utopias Project', as the opening quotation
implies, were resolutely positive in their answers to questions such as
these (Fung and Olin Wright, 2003a). And yet, a volatile mix of hope
and doubt currently surrounds citizen participation. Politicians from
traditions on the Left and on the Right declare faith in citizen capacity,

and call for citizen empowerment and partnerships in the development and delivery of public policy. They draw on experiments with citizens' juries, innovations in democratising local government, and on a range of novel practices in inclusive governance worldwide (Wainright, 2003). They see these as celebrations of democratic renewal and of a new contract between the governors and the governed. Others, including many who would deem themselves radicals, are not persuaded. They talk of cosmetic change, of efforts at legitimation and perhaps manipulation by governments (Cooke and Kothari, 2001). Equally unpersuaded, though rarely to be found in print, are some of those who have struggled to implement policy imperatives for participation, and have grown disillusioned. It is only a few, they complain, who come forward and those few are unrepresentative of the many. People who participate, they say, are often unrealistic in the demands that they make, or lacking in the competences that will enable them to understand the complexities and the constraints that those responsible for policy making and service delivery face. This final chapter confronts arguments such as these. On the basis of what is probably the most detailed ethnographic study to date, what can be concluded about the vexed questions of citizen capacity and capture? What messages can be gleaned about the pursuit of citizen participation initiatives; is it fashion, is it fantasy, or is it feasible?

The first section of the chapter concentrates on citizens themselves, on what it is that we can now say about what they bring to the deliberative arena and how they interact once there. We will highlight ways in which the findings of this study both confirm, but in important respects also challenge, previous work. The second section turns to the matter of hosting and designing citizen participation, teasing out what may be learned from the very active attempts made by the host organisation in this case study not only to encourage and shape deliberation itself, but also to position the results of citizen deliberation in relation to its many – not always enthusiastic – stakeholders. Questions about the place of initiatives such as these in the wider project known as democratic renewal are the subject matter of the final remarks.

The aim is to pursue the theme of pragmatic possibilities for the future. The chapter offers a series of messages about how to approach the question of 'citizen competence' and 'citizen capture' in ways that shift the terms of the debate, emphasising citizen potential and the power of the social, without minimising the challenges to be faced. At the same time, the chapter underlines the differences between local participatory initiatives and those, as here, involving citizens at the centre. All this takes us back, finally, to the context of change, and to visions – or the absence of clear visions – of the directions that 21st-century democracy might take. The 'real utopias' idea – the need for "hard-nosed proposals for pragmatically improving our institutions" rather than "vague utopian fantasies" (Olin Wright, 2003: vii) - remains in the forefront of the discussion.

Constructing the citizen

Writers on citizen participation often give a deeply pessimistic account of citizens themselves – they are negative about citizen motivation and willingness to engage, they doubt the competence and the ability of ordinary citizens to step back from their own experience and to consider the public good. Once in a deliberative arena, still in a negative vein, arguments continue that 'citizens don't …' and 'citizens can't …'. Such questioning of citizen capacities and competences has been a key factor, on the one hand, galvanising activists to design the experiments in deliberation represented in particular by citizens' juries, and, on the other, provoking the sceptical responses just outlined. To make progress in policy and practice, we need now to go beyond the simple polarisation of optimists and pessimists that pervades so much of this field. What can the case study of the NICE Citizens Council offer on this score?

Citizens engage

The first message that we draw from the present empirical research is this: *despite widespread assumptions about citizen apathy, it is possible to encourage large numbers of people to come forward for membership of a citizens' assembly.* Around 35,000 expressions of interest in a Citizens Council of NICE were received and over 4,000 people followed through with an application – responding to a challenge that was not about the immediacy of their own local services but about improving the NHS as a whole. What prompted them to act? Among the 30 people selected, wanting to make a contribution, helping to improve things, and a conviction that the public should be more involved in the services they funded and used, were the reasons cited in interviews. Comments such as these implied a concept of active responsibility as a citizen. Hoping to be stretched, to test themselves, and to do something new formed another cluster of reported motivators. What came over was a sense of unused capacity among citizens, of a hunger to learn and of a willingness to enter a collective arena which many admitted, with some trepidation, was something quite outside their previous experience. Hopes that they would 'make a difference' and in this instance noticeably 'improve the NHS' were not fulfilled in the time period in which we studied the Citizens Council, but the enthusiasm of virtually all the members remained apparent throughout. Two years on, and notwithstanding the difficulties of deliberation outlined in this book, their assessments remained largely positive. More than this, a substantial number of the original citizens councillors had plans to do more in future, to get involved in their local health trusts, for example.

Much credit for the high level of interest in this particular citizen participation initiative must be laid at the doors of the host organisation and the facilitation team. Already much in the public eye, NICE was able to orchestrate substantial high profile media attention. The Institute's work was complemented with active networking on the part of a team of facilitators with success in working with excluded groups. Just how much are portrayals of modern citizens as individualistic, cynical and disaffected or apathetic challenged by findings such as these? Should these results give pause both to generic narratives of the 'decline of the public' (Marquand, 2004), and to widespread arguments too that it is only direct self-interest, the promise of making a difference to one's own daily life, that will galvanise action? A recent independent inquiry into the state of democracy in Britain pointed in this direction:

> Contrary to much of the public debate around political disengagement, the British public are not apathetic. There is now a great deal of research evidence to show that very large numbers of citizens are engaged in community and charity work outside of politics. There is also clear evidence that involvement in pressure politics – such as signing petitions, supporting consumer boycotts, joining campaign groups – has been growing significantly for many years. In addition, research shows that interest in 'political issues' is high. (The POWER Inquiry, 2006: 15)

Plenty of questions must remain about 'how?', 'why?' and 'under what circumstances?', but there is enough here to conclude that the notion of citizens coming forward to participate is not an altogether utopian political vision. With political will, it can be nurtured and developed. The unhyphenated citizen may be a problematic identity with which to work (as indeed we argue below), but it is not an altogether empty category. In this instance, it proved entirely possible to call on what we might term background identities – collective commitments to 'our NHS', investments in notions of duty and of personal growth – to mobilise citizens and sustain their willingness to participate.

Citizen capacity or citizen potential? Changing the terms of the debate

Coming forward as individuals to participate is one thing, pulling off collective, and specifically deliberative, participation – a form of discussion that will tease out different positions, explore conflicting rationales for action and share ideas about what might constitute the common good – is another. We found that the amount of deliberation that took place in the Citizens Council rose over time and across the meetings observed; we also found that, overall, it remained very small. We argued that claims for deliberation, over the first two years of the Council, had not been met. What, in terms of practical policy, is to be concluded from this? Should the attempt simply be abandoned?

Here, drawing from an empirical example, is one suggestion about the dynamic of development of deliberation that strongly contests a pessimistic conclusion:

> Through the participatory process itself, people begin to perceive the needs of others, develop some solidarity, and conceptualize their own interests more broadly. Forced to confront their needs with others, arguments and reasons come to the fore ... in the Porto Alegre fora I studied, deliberation became more and more common over time as participants gained experience with public debate. (Abers, 2003: 206)

This account is drawn from an experiment in local participatory budget setting in Brazil and, formulated as one of a series of commentaries on this initiative and three others, it was presented as part of the Real Utopias Project mentioned earlier. It expresses what many see as the central dilemma of deliberation, namely that of overcoming self-interest. What is wanted, as the theory puts it, is not strategic action in pursuit of individual gain, but communicative action in pursuit of the good of the collective. Communicative action is a requirement, this response suggests, that over time will be met.

Something quite different was in play in the case we examined. It was not so much a question of the presence or absence of a capacity to transcend self-interest, but of the active creation of an expertise space for citizens as citizens – a firm set of grounds on which to engage with each other and with the questions set. In principle, Council members had a diversity of experiences to bring to bear on the matters under discussion. In practice, however, bringing lived experience into the debate was fraught with difficulty. Coming as 'ordinary people', just what could they bring? We showed how precarious was an identity constructed from 'common sense', a 'down to earth view' and a potentially 'bigger picture' than that of the professionals. We went on to demonstrate that citizens experimented with various culturally available speaking positions – the interrogator, for example, or the student. Different styles and speaking positions thus jostled with each other as citizens sought to find ways of making their interactions meaningful and relevant. In the process, focused questioning of witnesses, sustained discussion of their contributions and the teasing out of diverse potential positions in relation to the topic were casualties.

Compounding this difficulty was the sheer unfamiliarity of the situation, and the potential conflicts it might generate. Council members had expressed concerns in the initial interviews not only about what it was that would be required of them, but of how they would get on with each other, and how they would deal with any disagreements and conflicts that arose. The pressure, certainly at the outset, was to move quickly to a consensus rather than engage in the more risky pursuit of naming and exploring difference – seemingly a *reverse logic* compared with that outlined in the above quotation. Posing an abstract question for discussion exacerbated the difficulties and this argument is made in the body of the book. We would draw attention here, however, to the difference between involving citizens with an interest in a specific debate and involving unhyphenated citizens in a strategic debate about policy direction. This is by no means the first or the only exercise in involving citizens in a strategic debate in this way (see for example, Chapter Two, Box 2.2), but it does bring deliberation onto a terrain that has been less travelled both by activists and by theorists. Message two is therefore as follows: *in seeking to instate citizen deliberation in a context of handling strategic issues of policy direction, clarifying the grounds on which citizens are being asked to speak – creating, jointly with them, an expertise space in which they can call on familiar and emerging speaking positions – is fundamental.*

A great deal changed over the four meetings studied, as hosts and facilitators worked to find ways that would engage citizens more effectively. Different styles of presenting and assimilating information and of exploring value positions were tried. Role-plays, teasing out priorities by allocating paper money to photographed individuals, for example, were devices that were light-hearted and fun. They were also safe devices for starting to name and explore differences of values. Efforts at redesigning sessions, incorporating feedback from Council members themselves and moving away from reliance solely on the formal witness presentations, small groups and plenary debates on which the initial session had relied, were made and were appreciated by Council members. Less visible was the amount of behind-the-scenes support for members, both during the meetings and between them. We have tracked differences in emotional tone as citizens became more engaged. Council members began to make new sense of the task on which they had embarked, and to enjoy the challenge of making up and changing one's mind. And alongside elements of a 'reverse logic' of development compared with deliberation on local issues, familiarity, experience and experimentation with session design all served to enhance the potential for deliberative forms of interaction. Deliberation in the meetings of the Citizens Council, however, continued to occur in a fragile and fitful way. Message three then is that: *deliberation is a resource-intensive activity that needs continuing and imaginative forms of nurture, both by citizens and their hosts, in order to create an expertise space for citizens and to allow it to unfold.*

Nurturing deliberation remains more of an art than a science. Trainers were employed in three of the four experiments in participation in the Real Utopias Project. But what the agenda of training should be and how it might work to help people both to understand better their own self-interest and to work constructively with difference all remain unknown (Mansbridge, 2003:184–5). Our observation of the Citizens Council raised questions about ground rule setting and about what we called inclusive facilitation on the one hand and the more challenging facilitation for deliberation on the other. At present, it may be that "simply recognizing that closer examination is required and gathering cases in which that observation can take place are major advances" (Mansbridge, 2003: 187). Quite certainly, however, it is hard to imagine how, as some of the critics have been keen to suggest, the costs of deliberation could be cut by savings on citizen support. And without continuing attention to these matters there is a risk of reinstating the very orthodoxy of thinking that deliberation seeks to disrupt.

In sum, those who wish to bring citizens into the centre face challenges, some of which are the same as, and some different from, those seeking to take issues out to local citizens directly affected by them. In both cases, deliberation needs to be done knowingly, with recognition of the need for active support and nurture and the resource implications of this. But the argument being advanced here is much more than this. The key point for those who would create sites of citizen deliberation is not to talk of the 'capacity' or 'incapacity' of citizens as though this were also fixed or to assume that there are procedural solutions that will automatically generate deliberation. Instead, it is to consider ways of addressing citizen potential – creating what we have called an expertise space, an array of circumstances in which the relevance of diverse life experience can be brought into the arena and considered for its relevance to the topic in hand. And to talk of creating an expertise space in the way we are urging is not just to change the words, it is to change the terms of the debate, to transform the perception of citizens, and to acknowledge their potential both as individuals and in their social interaction with each other.

Diversity, inequality and oppositional discourses

Deliberation aspires to bring the full diversity of positions on a topic into a discussion arena and to give each of these a real chance to find expression. Only if this is done, and if the different positions are understood and acknowledged, can the discussion then move on to consider what might be proposed as the common good. We have already suggested that the expression of difference of opinion in a new and unfamiliar context such as the Citizens Council could be 'risky' for citizens. Where that difference counters conventionally accepted understandings of an issue, there is not only the risk of stating a position, but the challenge of finding words in which to articulate it that are both satisfying to oneself and accessible to others. Without access to languages of critique, opposition and resistance, members may be silenced and the rationale of deliberation put in jeopardy. For John Dryzek, prominent theorist in this field, enabling oppositional discourse is pivotal; the whole project of deliberative democracy is to "retrieve the critical voice" (Dryzek, 2000a: 30). Message four urges the overt recognition of this: *citizens are likely to find it difficult to initiate and pursue the discourses of opposition that deliberation seeks to make apparent; they need safe spaces and social practices that acknowledge and legitimate oppositional ideas in order to embark on this.*

Jane Mansbridge is again helpful in her comments on the Real Utopias experiments, succinctly capturing the theoretical dilemma, explaining its importance, and returning to the fraught question of self-interest. To focus on the common good is to make illegitimate what we have called strongly positioned statements, or, what she tellingly calls "assertions of self-interest". Yet the assertion of self-interest, as she points out, "helps one figure out oneself what one wants", and it helps one "in becoming understood (and respected) for what one wants and needs" (Mansbridge, 2003: 179). Our discussion in Chapter Two sought to accommodate this point by naming self-interest arguments as the necessary first step in a theory of the deliberative ideal. Citizens, however, need access to a route out of the dilemma of needing to express self-interest and yet feeling that it is not appropriate to do so. This is a particularly crucial point, since it is also the expression of self-interest that "helps unveil hegemonic understandings of the common good when those understandings have evolved to mask subtle forms of oppression" (Mansbridge, 2003: 179). This is a point we encountered in Chapter Two and elsewhere by reference to the work of Iris Marion Young and her discussions of the circumstances under which those who are subordinated and oppressed can be supported in finding expression for perspectives that go unrecognised by those in power. Without this, the putative benefits of diversity within the group will not be realised.

What can be said about self-interest and resistance to hegemonic thinking and the emergence of oppositional discourses on the basis of the ethnographic data from this study? Here, as Chapter Six has shown, were some of the most worrying results for those who would see citizens as deliberators and deliberative discussion as genuinely inclusive and generative of new ideas. One result of opacity about the grounds on which citizens could legitimately speak and of the pressures not to generate conflict was that, while differences of class, ethnicity, gender, disability and age were visible to all, the situation worked against the affirmation and exploration of such identities, and of the consequences that this might have for a fuller consideration of the topic under discussion. We saw this most dramatically in the clapping incident (Chapter Six), where all but two of the members strongly affirmed the notion of treating everyone 'the same'. We saw it also in the way in which efforts to devote a session to confronting notions of potential racism and sexism were questioned and resisted by the majority. And we saw it in the way in which the conclusion that avoiding accusations of ageism simply meant identical treatment for all quickly became a key and uncontested thread in the two meetings on the topic of age.

Citizens in this context did not feel themselves to be *representatives* of groups to which they belonged. But nor did they feel that they could, with ease, represent distinctive positions. Personal experience was too often dismissed as anecdote and as 'not relevant' to the topic. These dilemmas contributed to an inappropriate homogenising of citizens that we discussed in the last chapter.

How might 'safe spaces' be constructed here? Some of the answer lies in the techniques for nurturing identities as citizens noted above. Not enough thought has yet been given, however, to the subtleties of oppression, to the unconscious traces of hegemonic thinking that citizens themselves bring to the arena, as well as to the unacknowledged biases that hosts introduce in the framing of the question, the designing of sessions and the choice of witnesses. We saw glimpses of social practices that open up oppositional possibilities in the identity play that took place in performing set piece debates (see also Kulynych, 1997). We saw how the 'devil's advocate' role, introduced by the facilitators in later sessions, could help to enlarge citizens' horizons, challenge them to think differently and help them tease out the implications of such thinking. But we also stressed instances where deliberation took the form of collaborative enquiry (Extract 23) – another way perhaps of adjudicating between arguments and potentially transcending the terms of the official debate. Thus message five is: *citizens cannot be relied on as providing the sole source of oppositional ideas; different kinds and levels of critique need to be opened up and strongly legitimated as part of the process to which they are exposed.*

Deliberation as a process, then, needs further development. Citizens may well be motivated, resilient and willing to engage with each other. But this alone is not enough. Johnson (1998) is helpful in his pragmatic defence of deliberation and his argument that we must avoid making heroic assumptions on the one hand, and being ultra cynical on the other. Citizens, in other words need to be seen 'at normal size'. Pivotal to all this, also, however, is an acknowledgement of the power of the social. The ideas that emerge from a process of social interaction are not necessarily ones that any one participant would have reached alone. And if this is the case, we need to foster 'reflective solidarity' (Dean, 1996) – not the easy *solidarity in sameness* but the more difficult *solidarity in difference*, that demands a pause, requires respect for the other, and a willingness to reflect aloud and to shift positions. This is vital if the complexity and diversity of lived lives is to be brought in harness to a process of policy development. The power of the social is all too easily overlooked in a culture that celebrates the rational individual. Yet it is what underpins the very idea of deliberation.

If deliberation needs further development in order to work effectively for citizens, however, it also needs defending for its position in relation to other, more established and understood mechanisms of public policy making. The challenge for the host organisation in this case study was not only to find ways of creating deliberation *in situ* in the assembly, but also to defend the idea of deliberation and its place in pre-existing organisational arrangements that were themselves the subject of contestation. This is considered in the following section.

Questions of authority and independence

Advocates argue that deliberative assemblies bring new possibilities into the realm of political discussion. The inclusion of those not hitherto party to political debate, the replacement of dependency on experts with dialogue and the break with traditional adversarial stances, all, so the argument goes, point towards a politics capable of new ways of stating and realising collective values. We have examined and criticised one set of doubts on the grounds of citizen capacity. What then of the sceptics who come from another direction, arguing not so much that 'citizens can't...' but that 'those in power won't...'? Cohen and Rogers raise challenges for the citizen participation case studies in the Real Utopias Project on these grounds:

> The problem of generalizing deliberation is not that subordinate groups are unable to hold their own in deliberation, but that those with power advantages will not willingly submit themselves to the discipline of reason if that discipline presents large threats to their advantage. (Cohen and Rogers, 2003: 251)

Objections to deliberative assemblies on the grounds that the information to which they are exposed is unbalanced, that the agenda is controlled, or that they are mere 'talking shops' follow from this. Some who work in this field draw the conclusion that for deliberation to be worthwhile, it must give citizens themselves substantial agenda-setting power and be arranged and orchestrated by an independent body, not by an agency of the state (see, for example, Wakeford, 2002). The Citizens Council of NICE was a state-led initiative; it was the host organisation that set the questions to be discussed, who chose the witnesses and who decided what to do with the reports produced.

Entirely to dismiss the value of such initiatives on grounds that they are completely controlled by the powerful, however, is too harsh. Dryzek, strong proponent as we have seen of the need for critical and oppositional discourses in deliberative democracy, argues that if deliberation finds its "uniquely proper home" inside the institutional structures of liberal democracy, it will be "depleted of the resources it needs to reply to its critics more effectively" (Dryzek, 2000a: 3). But at the same time, he by no means rules out state-led initiatives:

> We should not give up on the possibility of authentic democracy within the confines of the state.... Sometimes it makes sense to highlight the state, sometimes civil society, and sometimes both. It all depends on the configuration of state imperatives and social movement interests, as well as the kind of inclusion that the state can offer to groups. (Dryzek, 2000a: 5)

Our data lend some support to such a position. As a state regulatory agency, NICE was nonetheless faced with a need repeatedly to 'explain' the Citizens Council to its varied stakeholders. The Institute struggled early on, for example, with just where the Council was to fit in the way its new, dialogic, consultative processes were configured (Davies, forthcoming). Members of its Partners Council, too, expressed unease, querying both the potential lack of independence for the citizens and where citizens' views were to fit alongside their own. Board meetings again meant defending the Council against criticism, and the impact workshops (Chapter Seven) brought both supporters and critics from in-house strongly into the frame. In all these cases, questions of the authoritativeness of outcomes from deliberation, and the defensibility and costs of the process, came onto the table for discussion.

What this indicates is that a deliberative assembly can have the capacity to disrupt established power relations. Disruption occurs regardless of whether or not its deliberations manage to produce disruptive thinking and regardless too of criticisms that may be levelled at its lack of independence. Deliberative assemblies can be expected to provoke resistance from established groups and the worldviews they espouse; deliberation's sponsors must expect actively to defend a deliberative assembly against its critics. Chapter Eight stressed the need for new kinds of theory to recognise that deliberation is never an island. Building on this now in terms of practical politics, message six is this: *deliberation always works in relation to pre-existing relations of power and of accountability; acknowledging this needs to be part of a shared rationale for embarking on it, and to be reflected in the ways in which the outcomes of deliberation are handled.*

Should the recommendations from a deliberation be binding on those who commission it? It was certainly never envisaged that this would be the case for the Citizens Council of NICE. The Council was to be advisory, it was to make reports to the Board, that would debate these and decide what action, if any, would then follow. There are, however, as we have noted at several points in this book, those who argue that recommendations emerging from a deliberative forum should be made mandatory. Close observation of the actuality of deliberation casts doubt on this. We would argue that any agreement that is reached through the imperfect and contingency-laden process that is likely to be deliberation in practice is better regarded as one resource among others for a democratic decision. Outcomes are better seen, in other words, as "necessarily conditional, tentative and revisable" (Johnson, 1998: 176; see also Lindeman, 2002). Council members themselves seemed to concur with this view. While some did raise concerns that the Council might end up as a 'cosmetic exercise', in the main, they were content to see their views being discussed and being taken into account. Some members, indeed, were distinctly uneasy about the responsibility that would be implied by anything more than this.

Another reason for placing deliberation as one resource among others is a matter of practical politics. The language of the inevitable debate that will surround the significance of a deliberative assembly and the fate of its recommendations is likely, in part at least, to be hostile to the structures and processes of deliberation. This was particularly clear in this case study at the point (discussed in Chapter Seven) where NICE initiated its in-house workshops as a means actively to integrate the work of the Council into its programmes of work and to consider what was to be done with its outputs. We demonstrated how the language of science and its assumptions surrounding acceptable evidence threatened to undermine the Council's output. We also showed that established consultation structures and routes of accountability left no obvious space in which the results of the Council's deliberations could be inserted. A deliberative assembly can never be designed in such a way as to guarantee the independence of thought that will generate alternatives to the *status quo*. Even where structures give it a degree of autonomy, hegemonic discourse will emerge both within the deliberative process and at the point of 'join' with other decision-making structures. Deliberative assemblies not only work in relation to existing authority structures, but to an important extent also always *within* those relations.

Arising from this, message seven is that: *the work of legitimating and integrating a deliberative assembly into already established institutional structures entails a confrontation both with the assumptions which underpin those structures, and with the language which has been developed to sustain them. Creating legitimate spaces to reflect on the alternative possibilities contained in these confrontations is an important condition for realising the hope for deliberation as a genuinely generative process.*

Developments in the period immediately following the completion of the research were a reminder of the contested political accountabilities in which NICE is enmeshed. The Institute was in the news in at least two high profile ways. First, there were demands that it should speed up the decision process on recommending drug approvals to the NHS. This was precipitated by media criticism about the continuing 'postcode lottery' during the time the Institute took to come to a decision on new drugs. Government pressure gave the Institute little option but to respond with revisions to its procedures (NICE, 2006). In this context, any arguments that might be advanced about placing the Citizens Council as another possible layer in the organisation's complex and time-consuming consultative process prior to decision, were pie in the political sky. Second, there was the outcry over Herceptin, a drug approved by NICE for late stage, but not for early stage, treatment in breast cancer. The plight of individual women generated much publicity; the Secretary of State seemingly overrode the Institute's guidance; cases were taken to the courts, critical coverage in the press continued and the matter was still very much ongoing as this book went to press. Both of these instances underline the points being made in this section, that deliberative assemblies are always nested in "background differences in power"(Cohen and Rogers, 2003: 250), and that what deliberation can do is give glimpses of alternative possibilities. Such possibilities, however, need to be, and will be, reflected on, reinforced or challenged in other spaces and places – importantly, but not exclusively, in the places designed to receive the results of deliberation and to mesh these with ongoing structures of accountability and decision. This brings us to some final remarks about the place of deliberative assemblies in the contemporary political project.

Deliberating in future

Writing in the context of the US, Cohen and Rogers (2003) position the experiments in participatory governance such as have been under discussion in this book as part of a post-socialist political project. Global social and economic shifts, they argue, have rendered state-centred regulatory strategies less plausible. These shifts have also brought uncertainties about socialism's commitment to egalitarian, participatory values and to the well-being of the working class. Thus a quest is now under way to find a new place for the state in new circumstances – a distinctive role in relation to asset redistribution perhaps (Bowles and Gintis, 1999; Paxton et al, 2006), but also a repositioning capable of acknowledging and fostering new forms of participatory citizenship. In an important passage on reframing values, these authors depict "a gradual emergence of a more inclusive, tolerant, cosmopolitan understanding of the political public", and they explain:

> An egalitarian-democratic project must respect the heterogeneity of reasonable political demands. But this heterogeneity immediately creates a political problem – how to achieve collective political focus, particularly among subordinate groups, on the achievement of any matter of shared concern. (Cohen and Rogers, 2003: 238)

The wide attraction of the process of deliberation and the creation of deliberative assemblies lies here.

All this plays out differently in different national contexts. We have seen, in the UK, that, while it was New Labour in power in the late 1990s that initiated a range of experiments in citizen participation, in the current repositioning of traditionally Left and Right parties, *all* are concerned about issues of disengagement and apathy, and all compete to declare the importance of direct citizen engagement in their programmes as they reach for political visions that transcend old categories and divisions. Debates about deliberation and democracy in political science, and debates about forms of practical democratic renewal across the political spectrum, have become thoroughly intertwined as both politicians and academics struggle to capture an understanding of a world of 'post-democracy' (Crouch, 2004), and design new political institutions to reflect its shifting economic and social contours.

There are a number of different threads to this. On the question of initiatives involving citizens that are designed to be deliberative, we have emphasised in this chapter, for example, the potentially different dynamics when citizens are invited to participate as locals, versus when they are asked to deliberate as *citizens at the centre*. We have discussed *state-led* assemblies versus those led by voluntary bodies. And we have seen earlier that alongside different designs for specifically deliberative forums (citizens panels, citizens' juries, deliberation days and so on), the rise of citizen participation has involved other more individualistic approaches – citizen engagement initiatives through holding consultation meetings, offering referendums and so on.

Seen from a perspective of democratic renewal, however, these various direct appeals to individuals as citizens to participate sit alongside calls for *organised stakeholders* to engage in more dialogue with each other and with governments. The global rise of social movements is reflected in a UK context in the emergence of a multiplicity of such stakeholders into the national political arena. Government restructuring has now written these into the political process, legitimating representation not only for trades unions, employers and business interests, but also for diverse publics organised around identities and single issues. Traditional lobby groups, new stakeholder interests and 'citizens' thus jostle for a place in political decision making. And this occurs alongside renewed debates about reforming the more familiar institutions of electoral democracy – be the proposals about new ways in which to vote or about the extension of eligibility to vote to previously excluded groups (The POWER Inquiry, 2006). These shifts are reflected academically in the popular work on participatory democracy discussed in Chapter One, in proposals, for example, on associative democracy (see Hirst, 1993; Cohen and Rogers, 1995), and in the calls for extension, for example, of stakeholder theory from its base in corporate and organisational contexts to economic and social governance more broadly (see, for example, Hutton, 1997).

Experiments in deliberation are thus both a reflection of, and a response to, unsettled times in the relations between governments and governed. Taking initiatives forward entails not only the challenges of creating and nurturing an expertise space for citizens, as discussed earlier in this chapter, but piloting the very idea of deliberative assemblies between the rocks of pre-established mechanisms of accountability. Perhaps the most detailed set of proposals on this issue at present, is that outlined in the Real Utopias Project, which gave this chapter its opening quotation. Fung and Olin Wright (2003b) begin from a commitment to what they call empowered participatory governance (EPG) – experiments in participation that focus on specific and tangible problems, that involve both officials and ordinary people affected by these problems, and that attempt to work deliberatively. For EPG to work, they argue, the institutions of government must adapt. Formal decision-making authority must be devolved to local units, new linkages of responsibility, resources and communication must connect different political levels with each other, and novel forms of state institution must be created to support and develop localised problem solving involving citizens. These proposals, they explain, acknowledge the dilemmas of what has gone before:

> Driven by the pragmatic imperative to find solutions that work, these new models reject both democratic centralism and strict decentralization as unworkable. The rigidity of the former leads it too often to disrespect local circumstance and intelligence and as a result it has a hard time learning from experience. Uncoordinated decentralization, on the other hand, isolates citizens into small units, surely a foolhardy measure for those who do not know how to solve a problem but suspect that others, somewhere else, do. (Fung and Olin Wright, 2003b: 21-2)

Theirs is thus not a straightforward argument for autonomous decentralisation, supporting those (discussed in the previous section) who would give authoritative decision-making power to a deliberative assembly. Instead, it is an argument for 'coordinated decentralisation', a concept which puts some flesh on the often vague calls for localism or people power that appear in party political programmes. Suggestive as these institutional design proposals are, however, they still, as commentators point out, constitute more of a normative vision than a practical theory specifying conditions under which such shifts can be instated (Cohen and Rogers, 2003: 249ff).

The challenge for those who seek to renew democracy is thus to provide multiple sites of deliberation, to locate these within policy development processes and to integrate all this both with stakeholder dialogue and with the institutions of majoritarian democracy. Electoral democracy, associative democracy and deliberative democracy all have a place in this — their clashing vocabularies and competing authorisations are vital resources through which political debate occurs. And deliberation, once an arcane debate among academics, has an integral place in this new project of governance. It has become central to current thinking about new directions for politics in the West.

The Citizens Council of NICE, studied in its first two years, then, was an ambiguous project, one full of dilemmas, whose discursive resolution was still being shaped as the study ended, and certainly could not have been predicted in advance. Creating a forum in which policy ideas can be digested and challenged, consciousness can be expanded, and hard choices can be addressed in terms of a notion of the common good, is a dream that continues to inspire politicians, academics and ordinary citizens themselves. To transform vision into practice it is more difficult than many are prepared to acknowledge. But it is not an impossible dream, and the directions in which to go to try to achieve it are perhaps a little clearer now than they were.

References

Abers, R.N. (2003) 'Reflections in what makes empowered participatory governance happen', in A. Fung and E. Olin Wright (eds) *Deepening democracy: Institutional innovations in empowered participatory governance*, London: Verso.

Appleby, J. and Coote, A. (2002) *Five-year health check: A review of government health policy 1997-2002*, London: King's Fund Policy Paper.

Armour, A. (1995) 'The citizens' jury model of public participation: a critical evaluation', in O. Renn, T. Webler and P. Wiedemann (eds) *Fairness and competence in citizen participation: Evaluating models for environmental discourse*, Dordrecht: Kluwer Academic Publishers.

Arnstein, S. (1969) 'A ladder of citizen participation', *Journal of the American Planning Association*, vol 35, no 4, pp 216-44.

Baggott, R., Allsop, J. and Jones, K. (2005) *Speaking for patients and carers: Health consumer groups and the policy process*, London: Palgrave.

Bang, H.P. and Dryberg, T.B. (2000) 'Governance, self-representation and democratic imagination', in M. Saward (ed) *Democratic innovation: Deliberation, representation and association*, London: Routledge.

Barber, B.R. (1984) *Strong democracy: Participatory politics for a new age*, London: California Press.

Barge, J.K. (1994) 'On interlinking language games: new opportunities for group communication research', *Communication Studies*, vol 45, pp 52-67.

Barge, J.K. (2002) 'Enlarging the meaning of group deliberation', in L.R. Frey (ed) *New directions in group communication*, Thousand Oaks, CA: Sage Publications.

Barnes, M. (1999) *Building a deliberative democracy: An evaluation of two citizens' juries*, London: IPPR.

Barnes, M. (2002) 'Bringing difference into deliberation? Disabled people, survivors and local governance', *Policy & Politics*, vol 30, no 3, pp 319-32.

Barnes, M. (2004) 'Affect, anecdote and diverse debates: user challenges to scientific rationality', in A. Gray and S. Harrison (eds) *Governing medicine: Theory and practice*, Maidenhead: Open University Press.

Barnes, M., Newman, J., Knops, A. and Sullivan, H. (2003) 'Constituting "the public" in public participation', *Public Administration*, vol 81, no 2, pp 379-99.

Bevir, M. (2004) 'Governance and interpretation: what are the implications of postfoundationalism?', *Public Administration*, vol 82, no 3, pp 605-25.

Bevir, M. and Rhodes, R.A.W. (2003) *Interpreting British governance*, London: Routledge.

Billig, M. (1987) *Arguing and thinking: A rhetorical approach to social psychology*, Cambridge: Cambridge University Press.

Billig, M. (1991) *Ideology and opinions: Studies in rhetorical psychology*, London: Sage Publications.

Billig, M. (2001) 'Discursive, rhetorical and ideological messages', in M. Wetherell, S. Taylor and S.J. Yates (eds) *Discourse theory and practice: A reader*, London: Sage Publications.

Billig, M., Condor, S., Edwards, D., Gane, M., Middleton, D. and Radley, A. (1988) *Ideological dilemmas*, London: Sage Publications.

Blair, T. (1998) *The third way: New politics for the new century*, London: Fabian Society.

Blowers, A. (2005) *Deliberative democracy and decision making for radioactive waste: A report for CoRWM*, London: DEFRA (www.corwm.org.uk).

Bourdieu, P. (1977) *Outline of a theory of practice*, Cambridge: Cambridge University Press.

Bourdieu, P. (1990) *Logic of practice*, Oxford: Polity.

Bowles, S. and Gintis, H. (1999) *Recasting egalitarianism: New rules for communities, states and markets*, London: Verso.

Budge, I. (2000) 'Deliberative democracy versus direct democracy – plus political parties!', in M. Saward (ed) *Democratic innovation: Deliberation, representation and association*, London: Routledge, pp 195-209.

Cabinet Office (1998a) *Quangos: Opening the doors*, London: Cabinet Office (Office of Public Services).

Cabinet Office (1998b) 'The listening government – People's Panel launched', Press release, 29 January.

Cabinet Office (2002) *Public bodies: Opening up public appointments, 2002–2005* (www.cabinet-office.gov.uk).

Cabinet Office (2004) *Code of good practice on consultation* (www.cabinetoffice.gov.uk/regulation/consultation/code.htm).

Cameron, D. (2001) *Working with spoken discourse*, London: Sage Publications.

Charlton, B.G. (2000) 'The new management of scientific knowledge in medicine', in A. Miles, J.R. Hampton and B. Hurwitz (eds) *NICE, CHI and the NHS reforms: Enabling excellence or imposing control?*, London: Aesculapius Press, pp 13-32.

Charlton, B.G. and Miles, A. (1998) 'The rise and fall of EBM', *QJM*, vol 91, pp 371-4.

Cheyne, C. and Comrie, M. (2002) 'Enhanced legitimacy for local authority decision making: challenges, setbacks and innovation', *Policy & Politics*, vol 30, no 4, pp 469-82.

Chia, R. (2000) 'Discourse analysis as organizational analysis', *Organization*, vol 7, no 3, pp 513-18.

Church, K. (1996) 'Beyond "bad manners": the power relations of "consumer participation" in Ontario's community mental health system', *Canadian Journal of Community Mental Health*, vol 15, pp 27-44.

Cicourel, A.V. (1981) 'Notes on the integration of micro and macro levels of analysis', in K. Knorr-Cetina and A.V. Cicourel (eds) *Advances in social theory and methodology: Towards an integration of micro and macro sociologies*, Boston, MA: Routledge and Kegan Paul, pp 51-80.

Clarke, R. (2002) *New democratic processes: Better decisions, stronger democracy*, London: IPPR.

Cohen, J. (1998) 'Democracy and liberty', in Elster, J. (ed) *Deliberative Democracy*, Cambridge: Cambridge University Press.

Cohen, J. and Rogers, J. (1995) *Associations and democracy*, London: Verso.

Cohen, J. and Rogers, J. (2003) 'Power and reasons', in A. Fung and E. Olin Wright (eds) *Deepening democracy: Institutional innovations in empowered participatory governance*, London: Verso.

Collins, H.M. and Evans, R. (2002) 'The third wave of science studies: studies of expertise and experience', *Social Studies of Science*, vol 32, no 2, pp 235-96.

Cooke, B. and Kothari, U. (eds) (2001) *Participation: The new tyranny?*, London: Zed Books.

Coote, A. and Lenaghan, J. (1997) *Citizens' juries: Theory into practice*, London: IPPR.

Coulter, A. (2002) *The autonomous patient: Ending paternalism in medical care*, London: The Nuffield Trust/The Stationery Office.

Coulter, A. and Ham, C. (2000) *Global challenge of health care rationing*, Buckingham: Open University Press.

Crosby, N. (1995) 'Citizens juries: one solution for difficult environmental questions', in O. Renn, T. Webler and P. Wiedemann (eds) *Fairness and competence in citizen participation: Evaluating models for environmental discourse*, Dordrecht: Kluwer Academic Publishers.

Crouch, C. (2004) *Post-democracy*, Cambridge: Polity Press.

CSJ (Commission on Social Justice) (1994) *Social justice: Strategies for national renewal*, London: Vintage.

Cutler, T. and Waine, B. (2000) 'Managerialism reformed? New Labour and public sector management', *Social Policy and Administration*, vol 34, no 3, pp 318-32.

Davies, C. (2001) *Lay involvement in professional reputation: A study of public appointment-holders in the health field*, Milton Keynes: Open University, School of Health and Social Welfare.

Davies, C. (2003) 'Introduction: a new workforce in the making?', in C. Davies (ed) *The future health worker*, London: Palgrave.

Davies, C. (forthcoming) 'Grounding governance in dialogue? Discourse, practice and the potential for a new public sector organisational forum', *Public Administration*.

Davies, C., Wetherell, M., Barnett, E. and Seymour-Smith, S. (2005) *Opening the box: Evaluating the Citizens Council of NICE*, Report prepared for the National Co-ordinating Centre for Research Methodology, NHS R&D Programme (www.pcpoh.bham.ac.uk/publichealth/nccrm/publications.htm).

Davies, S., Elizabeth, S., Hanley, B., New, B. and Sang, B. (1998) *Ordinary wisdom: Reflections on an experiment in citizenship and health*, London: King's Fund Publishing.

Dean, J. (1996) *Solidarity of stranger: Feminism after identity politics*, London: University of California Press.

DETR (Department of the Environment, Transport and the Regions) (1998) *Modern local government: In touch with the people*, Cm 4014, London: The Stationery Office.

DH (Department of Health) (1997) *The new NHS: Modern, dependable*, Cm 3807, London: The Stationery Office.

DH (1998) *A first class service: Quality in the new NHS*, London: DH.

DH (2000) *The NHS Plan: A plan for investment. A plan for reform*, London: DH.

DH (2003) *Strengthening accountability: Involving patients and the public*, Policy Guidance on the Statutory Duties, Section II, Health and Social Care Act, 2001, London: DH.

DH (2004) *Patient and public involvement in health: The evidence for policy implementation: A summary of the results of the Health in Partnership Research Programme*, London: DH.

Dienel, P.C. and Renn, O. (1995) 'Planning cells: a gateway to "fractal" mediation', in O. Renn, T. Webler and P. Wiedemann (eds) *Fairness and competence in citizen participation: Evaluating models for environmental discourse*, Dordrecht: Kluwer Academic Publishers.

Dolan, P., Cookson, R. and Ferguson, B. (1999) 'Effect of discussion and deliberation on the public's views of priority-setting in health care: focus group study', *British Medical Journal*, vol 318, pp 916-19.

Dryzek, J. (2000a) *Deliberative democracy and beyond: Liberals, critics, contestations*, Oxford: Oxford University Press.

Dryzek, J. (2000b) 'Discursive democracy vs liberal constitutionalism', in M. Saward (ed) *Democratic innovation: Deliberation, representation vs association*, London: Routledge.

Dunkerley, D. and Glasner, P. (1998) 'Empowering the public? Citizens' juries and the new genetics technologies', *Critical Public Health*, vol 8, no 3, pp 181-92.

Eckert, P. (2000) *Linguistic variation as social practice*, Oxford: Blackwell.

Edelenbos, J. and Klijn, E.-H. (2004) 'The impact of organizational arrangements in the outcomes of interactive decision-making in the Netherlands', ESRC/EPSRC Colloquium 'Governance and performance', University of Birmingham, March.

Edwards, D. and Potter, J. (1992) *Discursive psychology*, London: Sage Publications.

Elgood, J. and Mountford, S. (2000) *Public perceptions of the ministerial appointments process: Combined qualitative and quantitative report*, London: MORI (www.ocpa.gov.uk).

Elster, J. (ed) (1998) *Deliberative democracy*, Cambridge: Cambridge University Press.

Fairclough, N. (2000) *New Labour, new language?*, London: Routledge.

Farrell, C. (2004) *Patient and public involvement in health: The evidence for policy implementation*, London: DH.

Fishkin, J.S. (1995) *The voice of the people: Public opinion and democracy*, New Haven, CT: Yale University Press.

Fishkin, J.S. and Luskin, R.C. (2000) 'The quest for deliberative democracy', in M. Saward (ed) *Democratic innovation: Deliberation, representation and association*, London: Routledge.

Fitch, K. (2001) 'The ethnography of speaking: Sapir/Whorf, Hymes and Moerman', in M. Wetherell, S.J. Taylor and S.J. Yates (eds) *Discourse theory and practice: A reader*, London: Sage Publications, pp 57-64.

Fung, A. and Olin Wright, E. (eds) (2003a) *Deepening democracy: Institutional innovations in empowered participatory governance*, London: Verso.

Fung, A. and Olin Wright, E. (2003b) 'Thinking about empowered participatory governance', in A. Fung and E. Olin Wright (eds) *Deepening democracy: Institutional innovations in empowered participatory governance*, London: Verso.

Geertz, C. (1973) *The interpretation of cultures*, New York, NY: Basic Books.

Gergen, K. (1985) 'The social constructionist movement in modern psychology', *American Psychologist*, vol 40, pp 266-75.

Giddens, A. (1979) *Central problems in social theory*, London: Macmillan.

Giddens, A. (1991) *Modernity and self-identity*, Cambridge: Polity Press.

Giddens, A. (1994) *Beyond Left and Right: The future of radical politics*, Cambridge: Polity Press.

Giddens, A. (1998) *The third way: The renewal of social democracy*, Oxford: Blackwell/Polity Press.

Giddens, A. (2000) *The third way and its critics*, Oxford: Blackwell/Polity Press.

Goffman, E. (1974) *Frame analysis*, London: Harper and Row.

Gopal, K. (1999) 'Damage control', *Pharmaceutical Executive*, November, p 35.

Gopal, K. (2001) 'NICE says no to MS', *Pharmaceutical Executive*, September, p 26.

Griffiths, L. (2002) 'Humour as resistance to professional dominance in community mental health teams', in S. Taylor (ed) *Ethnographic research: A reader*, London: Sage Publications.

Griffiths, R. (1983) *NHS management inquiry: Report to the Secretary of State for Social Services*, London: DHSS.

Gulland, A. (2002) 'NICE proposals for Citizens Council condemned by patients', *British Medical Journal*, vol 325, issue 7361, p 406, 24 August.

Gutman, A. and Thompson, D. (2002) 'Deliberative democracy beyond process', *The Journal of Political Philosophy*, vol 10, no 2, pp 153-74.

Habermas, J. (1984) *Theory of communicative action: Vol 1: Reason and rationalisation of society*, Boston, MA: Beacon Press.

Habermas, J. (1987) *Theory of communicative action: Vol 2: System and lifeworld*, Boston, MA: Beacon Press.

Habermas, J. (1996) 'Three normative models of democracy', in S. Benhabib (ed) *Democracy and difference: Contesting the boundaries of the political*, Princeton, NJ: Princeton University Press.

Ham, C. and Robert, G. (eds) (2003) *Reasonable rationing: International experience of priority setting in health care*, Maidenhead: Open University Press.

Harrison, S. and Mort, M. (1998) 'Which champions, which people? Public and user involvement in health care as a technology of legitimation', *Social Policy & Administration*, vol 32, no 1, pp 60-70.

Hayden, C. and Boaz, A. (2000) *Making a difference: Better Government for Older People*, Evaluation Report, Coventry: University of Warwick, Local Government Centre.

Hendriks, C. (2002) 'Institutions of deliberative democratic processes and interest groups: roles, tensions and incentives', *Australian Journal of Public Administration*, vol 61, no 1, pp 64-75.

Hewes, D.E. (1996) 'Small group communication may not influence decision making: an amplification of socio-ego-centristic theory', in R.Y. Hirokawa and M.S. Poole (eds) *Communication and group decision making*, Thousand Oaks, CA: Sage Publications.

Hirst, P. (1993) *Associative democracy: New forms of economic and social governance*, Cambridge: Polity Press.

Hirst, P. (1994) *Associative democracy*, Cambridge: Polity Press.

Hirst, P. and Khilnani, S. (eds) (1996) *Reinventing democracy*, Oxford: Blackwell.

Hodge, S. (2005) 'Discourse and power: a case study in service user involvement', *Critical Social Policy*, vol 83, no 25, pp 164-79.

Hogg, C. (1999) *Patients, power and politics: From patients to citizens*, London: Sage Publications.

Hogg, C. and Williamson, C. (2001) 'Whose interests do lay people represent? Towards an understanding of the role of lay people as members of committees', *Health Expectations*, vol 4, pp 2-9.

Hogwood, B. and Gunn, L. (1984) *Policy analysis for the real world*, London: Oxford University Press.

House of Commons Select Committee on Public Administration (1999) *Minutes of evidence, examination of witnesses*, Tuesday 30 November.

House of Commons Select Committee on Public Administration (2001a) *Sixth Report: Innovations in citizen participation in government.*

House of Commons Select Committee on Public Administration (2001b) *First Report: Public participation: Issues and innovations: The government's response to the Committee's Sixth Report of Session 2000–01* (www.publications.parliament.uk/pa/cm200102/cmselect/cmpubadm/334/33403.htm).

House of Lords Select Committee on Science and Technology (2000) *Science and society*, London: House of Lords, 23 February.

Husband, C. (1986) 'The concepts of attitude and prejudice in the mystification of "race" and "racism"', Paper presented at the BPS Social Psychology Section Annual Conference, University of Sussex.

Hutchins, E. and Klausen, T. (2002) 'Distributed cognition in an airline cockpit', in S. Taylor (ed) *Ethnographic research: A reader*, London: Sage Publications.

Hutton, W. (1995) *The state we're in*, London: Vintage.

Hutton, W. (1997) *The state to come*, London: Vintage.

Johnson, J. (1998) 'Arguing for deliberation: some sceptical considerations', in J. Elster (ed) *Deliberative democracy*, Cambridge: Cambridge University Press.

Jowell, T. (2005) *Tackling the 'poverty of aspiration' through rebuilding the public realm*, London: Demos.

Kashefi, E. and Mort, M. (2004) 'Grounded citizens' juries: a tool for health activism?', *Health Expectations*, vol 7, no 4, pp 290-302.

Kennedy Report (2001) *The Report of the Public Inquiry into Children's Heart Surgery at the Bristol Royal Infirmary 1984-1995*, Cm 5207(1), London: The Stationery Office.

Klein, R. (2001) *The new politics of the NHS* (4th edn), London: Prentice Hall.

Kulynych, J. (1997) 'Performing politics: Foucault, Habermas, and postmodern participation', *Polity*, vol 30, no 2, pp 315-46.

Laclau, E. and Mouffe, C. (1987) 'Post-Marxism without apologies', *New Left Review*, vol 166, pp 79-106.

Lave, J. and Wenger, E. (1991) *Situated learning: Legitimate, peripheral participation*, Cambridge: Cambridge University Press.

LGMB (Local Government Management Board) (1996) *Citizens' juries in local government: Report for LGMB on the pilot projects*, London: LGMB.

Lindeman, M. (2002) 'Opinion quality and policy preferences in deliberative research', in M.X. Delli Carpini, L. Huddy and R.Y. Shapiro (eds) *Political decision-making, deliberation and participation*, Amsterdam and London: JAI Press.

Lister, R. (2001) 'New Labour: a study in ambiguity from a position of ambivalence', *Critical Social Policy*, vol 21, no 4, pp 425-47.

Lowndes, V., Pratchett, L. and Stoker, G. (2001a) 'Trends in public participation: Part 1 – Local government perspective', *Public Administration*, vol 79, no 1, pp 205-22.

Lowndes, V., Pratchett, L. and Stoker, G. (2001b) 'Trends in public participation: Part 2 – Citizens' perspectives', *Public Administration*, vol 79, no 2, pp 445-55.

Lyman, P. (1981) 'The politics of anger: on silence, ressentiment and political speech', *Socialist Review*, vol 11, no 3, pp 55-74.

McIver, S. (1998) *Healthy debate? An independent evaluation of citizens' juries in health settings*, London: King's Fund Publishing.

Mansbridge, J. (2003) 'Practice-thought practice', in A. Fung and E. Olin Wright (eds) *Deepening democracy: Institutional innovations in empowered participatory governance*, London: Verso.

Marquand, D. (2004) *Decline of the public: The hollowing-out of citizenship*, Cambridge: Polity Press.

Maybin, J. (2001) 'Language, struggle and voice: the Bakhtin/Voloshinov writings', in M.S. Wetherell, S.J. Taylor and S.J. Yates (eds) *Discourse theory and practice: A reader*, London: Sage Publications.

Mendelberg, T. (2002) 'The deliberative citizen: theory and evidence', in M.X. Delli Carpini, L. Huddy and R.Y. Shapiro (eds) *Political decision-making, deliberation and participation*, Amsterdam and London: JAI Press.

Meyers, R.A. and Brashers, D.E. (2002) 'Rethinking traditional approaches to argument in groups', in L.R. Frey (ed) *New directions in group communication*, Thousand Oaks, CA: Sage Publications.

Midden, C.J.H. (1995) 'Direct participation in macro-issues: a multiple group approach. an analysis and critique of the Dutch national debate on energy policy; fairness, competence, and beyond', in O. Renn, T. Webler and P. Wiedemann (eds) *Fairness and competence in citizen participation: Evaluating models for environmental discourse*, Dordrecht: Kluwer Academic Publishers.

Miles, A., Hampton, J.R. and Hurwitz, B. (eds) *NICE, CHI and the NHS reforms: Enabling excellence or imposing control?*, London: Aesculapius Press, pp 13-32.

Morson, G.S. and Emerson, C. (1990) *Mikhail Bakhtin: Creation of a prosaics*, Stanford, CA: Stanford University Press.

Mullen, P.M. (1999) 'Public involvement in health care priority setting: an overview of methods for eliciting values', *Health Expectations*, vol 2, pp 222-34.

Mumpower, J.L. (1995) 'The Dutch Study Groups revisited', in O. Renn, T. Webler and P. Wiedemann (eds) *Fairness and competence in citizen participation: Evaluating models for environmental discourse*, Dordrecht: Kluwer Academic Publishers.

NHSME (National Health Service Management Executive) (1992) *Local voices: The views of local people in commissioning for health*, London: NHSME.

Newman, J. (2001) *Modernising governance: New Labour, policy and society*, London: Sage Publications.

Newman, J. (2005) *Remaking governance: Peoples, politics and the public sphere*, Bristol: The Policy Press.

NICE (2006) *Selection of topics*, Consultation Paper, March.

Oetzel, J.G. (2001) 'The effects of culture and cultural diversity on communication in work groups', in L.R. Frey (ed) *New directions in group communication*, Thousand Oaks, CA: Sage Publications.

Olin Wright, E. (2003) 'Preface: the Real Utopias Project', in A. Fung and E. Olin Wright (eds) *Deepening democracy: Institutional innovations in empowered participatory governance*, London: Verso.

Parkinson, J. (2004a) 'Hearing voices: negotiating representation claims in public deliberation', *Political Studies Association*, vol 6, pp 370-88.

Parkinson, J. (2004b) 'Why deliberate? The encounter between deliberation and the new public managers', *Public Administration*, vol 82, no 2, pp 377-95.

Pateman, C. (1976) *Participation and democratic theory*, Cambridge: Cambridge University Press.

Pavitt, C. and Johnson, K.K. (1999) 'An examination of the coherence of group discourse', *Communication Research*, vol 26, no 3, pp 303-21.

Paxton, W., White, S. and Maxwell, D. (2006) *The citizen's stake: Exploring the future of universal asset policies*, Bristol: The Policy Press.

Peck, E. (1998) 'Integrity, ambiguity or duplicity? NHS consultation with the public', *Health Services Management Research*, vol 4, pp 201-10.

PEALS (2003) *Teach yourself citizens juries: A handbook by the DIY Jury Steering Group*, Newcastle: University of Newcastle.

Petts, J. (2001) 'Evaluating the Effectiveness of deliberative processes: waste management case-studies', *Journal of Environmental Planning and Management*, vol 44, no 2, pp 207-26.

Phillips, A. (1995) *The politics of presence*, Oxford: Clarendon Press.

Pickard, S. (1998) 'Citizenship and consumerism in health care: a critique of citizens' juries', *Social Policy & Administration*, vol 32, no 3, pp 226-44.

Polkinghorne, D.E. (1988) *Narrative knowing and the human sciences*, Albany, NY: State University of New York Press.

Potter, J. and Wetherell, M. (1987) *Discourse and social psychology: Beyond attitudes and behaviour*, London: Sage Publications.

Powell, M. (2000) 'New Labour and the third way in the British welfare state: a new and distinctive approach?', *Critical Social Policy*, vol 20, no 1, pp 39-60.

Pratchett, L. (1999) 'New fashions in public participation: towards greater democracy?', *Parliamentary Affairs*, vol 52, no 4, pp 616-33.

Price, D. (2000) 'Choices without reasons: citizens juries and policy evaluation', *Journal of Medical Ethics*, vol 26, pp 272-6.

Prior, D., Stewart, J. and Walsh, K. (1995) *Citizenship: Rights, community and participation*, London: Pearson.

Putnam, R. (2000) *Bowling alone: The collapse and revival of American community*, London: Simon and Schuster.

Quennell, P. (2001) 'Getting their say, or getting their way? Has participation strengthened the patient "voice" in the national institute for clinical excellence?', *Journal of Management in Medicine*, vol 15, no 3, pp 202-19.

Rawlins, M.D. and Culyer, A.J. (2003) *Scientific and social value judgements*, London: National Institute for Clinical Excellence.

Rawls, J. (1971) *A theory of justice*, Cambridge, MA: Harvard University Press.

Rawls, J. (1997) 'The idea of public reason revisited', *University of Chicago Law Review*, vol 64, pp 765-807.

Reed, M. (2004) 'Getting real about organisational discourse', in D. Grant, C. Hardy, C. Osweick and L. Putnam (eds) *The SAGE handbook of organisational discourse*, London: Sage Publications.

Reeves, F. (1983) *British racial discourse*, Cambridge: Cambridge University Press.

Renn, O., Webler, T. and Wiedemann, P. (eds) (1995) *Fairness and competence in citizen participation: Evaluating models for environmental discourse*, Dordrecht: Kluwer Academic Publishers.

Ritchie, J. and Spencer, L. (1994) 'Qualitative data analysis for applied policy research', in A. Bryman and R. Burgess (eds) *Analysing qualitative data*, London: Routledge.

Rowe, M. and Devaney, C. (2003) 'Partnership and the governance of regeneration', *Critical Social Policy*, vol 23, no 3, pp 375-96.

Sackett, D., Richardson, W.S., Rosenberg, W. and Haynes, P. (1996) *Evidence-based medicine*, London: Churchill-Livingstone.

Sanders, L. (1997) 'Against deliberation', *Political Theory*, vol 25, pp 347-476.

Saward, M. (ed) (2000) *Democratic innovation: Deliberation, representation and association*, London: Routledge.

Schatzki, T.R., Knorr-Cetina, K.D. and von Savigny, E. (eds) (2001) *The practice turn in contemporary theory*, London: Routledge.

Secretary of State for Health (2001) *Learning from Bristol: The Report of the Public Inquiry into Children's Heart Surgery at the Bristol Royal Infirmary*, Cm 5207(1), London: The Stationery Office.

Secretary of State for Health (2006) Statement to the House, 1 March 2006, *Hansard,* col 26WS.

Smith, G. (2001) 'Taking deliberation seriously: institutional design and green politics', *Environmental Politics*, vol 10, no 3, pp 72-93.

Smith, G. (2003) *Deliberative democracy and the environment*, London: Routledge.

Smith, G. (2005) *Beyond the ballot: 57 democratic innovations from around the world. A report for the Power Inquiry*, London: POWER Inquiry.

Smith, G. and Wales, C. (1999) 'The theory and practice of citizens' juries', *Policy & Politics*, vol 27, no 3, pp 295-308.

Smith, G. and Wales, C. (2000) 'Citizens' juries and deliberative democracy', *Political Studies*, vol 48, pp 51-65.

Squires, J. (1998) 'In different voices: deliberative democracy and aesthetic politics', in J. Goode and I. Velody (eds) *The politics of postmodernity*, Cambridge: Cambridge University Press.

Stewart, J. (1996) 'Innovation in democratic practice in local government', *Policy & Politics*, vol 24, no 1, pp 29-41.

Stewart, J., Kendall, E. and Coote, A. (1994) *Citizen's juries*, London: IPPR.

Stirling, A. (2005) 'Opening up or closing down? Analysis, participation and power in the social appraisal of technology', in M. Leach, I. Scoones and B. Wynne (eds) *Science and citizens: Globalization and the challenge of engagement*, London: Zed Books.

Stokes, S.C. (1998) 'Pathologies of deliberation', in J. Elster (ed) *Deliberative democracy*, Cambridge: Cambridge University Press, pp 123-39.

Stokkom, B. (2005) 'Deliberative group dynamics: power, status and affect in interactive policy making', *Policy & Politics*, vol 33, no 3, pp 387-409.

Taylor, J.R. and Every, E.J. (2000) *The emergent organisation: Communication as its site and surface*, Mahwah, NJ: Lawrence Erlbaum.

The POWER Inquiry (2006) *Power to the people. The report of POWER: An independent enquiry into Britain's democracy*, York: York Publishing Services.

Thompson, S. and Hoggett, P. (2001) 'The emotional dynamics of deliberative democracy', *Policy & Politics*, vol 29, no 3, pp 351-63.

Tritter, J. (2006: forthcoming) 'The snakes and ladders of user involvement: moving beyond Arnstein'.

Tsoukas, H. and Chia, R. (2002) 'On organizational becoming: rethinking organizational change', *Organization Science*, vol 13, no 5, pp 567-82.

van Dijk, T. (1980) *Macrostructures*, Hillsdale, NJ: Lawrence Erlbaum.

Vivian, M. (2004) *'Getting over the wall': How the NHS is improving the patient's experience*, London: DH (www.dh.gov.uk/assetRoot/04/09/08/66/04090866.pdf).

Wainright, H. (2003) *Reclaim the state: Experiments in popular democracy*, London: Verso.

Wakeford, T. (2002) 'Citizens juries: a radical alternative for social research', *Social Research Update*, University of Surrey, Issue 37.

Walshe, K. (2002) 'The rise of regulation in the NHS', *British Medical Journal*, vol 324, pp 967-70.

Warde, A. (2004) *Practice and field: Revising Bourdieusian concepts*, CRIC Discussion Paper No 65, Manchester: University of Manchester.

Watson, W.E., Kumar, K. and Michaelson, L.K. (1993) 'Cultural diversity's impact on interaction process and performance: comparing homogeneous and diverse task groups', *Academy of Management Journal*, vol 36, pp 590-602.

Webler, T. (1995) '"Right" discourse in citizen participation: an evaluative yardstick', in O. Renn, T. Webler and P. Wiedemann (eds) *Fairness and competence in citizen participation: Evaluating models for environmental discourse*, Dordrecht: Kluwer Academic Publishers.

Webster, C. (1998) *The National Health Service: A political history*, Oxford: Oxford University Press.

Weick, K.E. (1979) *The social psychology of organising* (2nd edn), Reading, MA: Addison-Wesley.

Weick, K.E. (1995) *Sensemaking in organisations*, London: Sage Publications.

Weick, K.E. (2004) 'A bias for conversation: acting discursively in organisations', in D. Grant, C. Hardy, C. Oswick and L. Putnam (eds) *The SAGE handbook of organisational discourse*, London: Sage Publications.

Wenger, E. (1999) *Communities of practice: Learning, meaning and identity*, Cambridge: Cambridge University Press.

Wetherell, M. and Potter, J. (1992) *Mapping the language of racism: Discourse and the legitimation of exploitation*, London and New York, NY: Harvester Wheatsheaf and Columbia University Press.

Wetherell, M., Taylor, S. and Yates, S.J. (2001a) *Discourse theory and practice*, London: Sage Publications.

Wetherell, M., Taylor, S. and Yates, S.J. (2001b) *Discourse as data*, London: Sage Publications.

Williams, M. (2004) 'Discursive democracy and New Labour: five ways in which decision-makers manage citizen agendas in public participation initiatives', *Sociological Research Online*, vol 9, no 3 (www.socresonline.org.uk).

Wilsdon, J. and Willis, R. (2004) *See-through science: Why public engagement needs to move upstream*, London: Demos.

Wood, B. (2000) *Patient power?*, Buckingham: Open University Press.

Wynne, B. (2005) 'Risk as globalising "democratic" discourses? Framing subjects and citizens', in M. Leach, I. Scoones and B. Wynne (eds) *Science and citizens*, London: Zed Books.

Young, I.M. (1989) 'Polity and group difference: a critique of the ideal of universal citizenship', *Ethics*, vol 99, pp 250-74.

Young, I.M. (1990) *Justice and the politics of difference*, Princeton, NJ: Princeton University Press.

Young, I.M. (1996) 'Communication and the other: beyond deliberative democracy', in S. Benhabib (ed) *Democracy and difference: Contesting the boundaries of the political*, Princeton, NJ: Princeton University Press.

Young, I.M. (2000) *Inclusion and democracy*, Oxford: Oxford University Press.

Study design and methods

The empirical research reported in this book is based on a study commissioned by the NHS R&D Methodology Programme with the stated aim of providing information for policy makers on how best to make use of citizens' time when members of the public are invited to discuss complex issues. A detailed final report of this evaluation study was prepared (Davies et al, 2005) and is available on the Methodology Programme website (www.pcpoh.bham.ac.uk/publichealth/nccrm/). An effective research evaluation of a complex policy initiative puts demands on the researchers to familiarise themselves with the context in which the new development is taking place and to develop an awareness of the intentions, hopes and fears of all parties. The various strands of work required by the commissioners were therefore assembled into three component parts. At the core was an *ethnographic study*, consisting of observations of the Citizens Council in session. There was an *organisation study*, which aimed to comment on the climate in which the Citizens Council initiative had arisen and to monitor its development. There was also *the study of the citizens themselves*, which explored the significance of the initiative from their point of view and examined the challenges, intended and unintended, that it generated for them. This appendix gives further details on each of these.

All aspects of the study were explained to Citizens Council members at their induction meeting in November 2002 and explicit consent was sought both for the ethnographic study and for interviews in a face-to-face setting. We worked in accordance with the British Psychological Society's Code of Conduct for psychologists conducting research with human participants in inviting all Citizens Council members to give written consent to participation in the project. Initially, 29 of the 30 original members gave this consent. However, in the fourth meeting, where consent forms were secured from the 10 new recruits to the Council, consent was also forthcoming from the one remaining member from the original group. Participants were advised that they could withdraw their data at any point. They were kept informed at all stages of the process and we debriefed them at the fourth meeting. Although the names of Citizens Council members are in the public domain, we have used pseudonyms in all project outputs including this book in order to protect the identity of each member of the Citizens Council in discussions of the dynamics of the Council and in commenting on its overall performance. Written consents were similarly secured from staff of the Institute and others for individual interviews. All data have been kept securely following data protection guidelines.

Ethnographic study

The funders had explicitly requested an ethnographic study and had indicated that it should form the major component of the work. The design developed by the team sought to capture the details of the actual practice in Citizens Council meetings through the analysis of transcripts from video-recordings provided by a professional camera crew, familiar with the demands of filming discretely. The first three meetings were to be analysed in depth with the fourth serving as a check for the analysis.

Ethnography involves a 'thick description' (Geertz, 1973) of social life. It aims to provide a closely observed and objective account of what actually happened rather than to rely on 'received views' from participants. This is important for two reasons. First, the alternative of relying on memories and reconstructions of an event is rarely reliable. An 'agreed view' quickly develops for something as complex as a Citizens Council meeting, and this snapshot might well be very misleading. Second, it is entirely possible that detailed attention to a process on the ground will reveal new and more productive ways of achieving the required result when compared with reliance on responses to preset questions or pre-established evaluation criteria.

Among ethnographic researchers there is now a growing move away from methods based on observation notes and impressions and towards the creation of a more robust record of interactions using video and audio techniques (Griffiths, 2002; Hutchins and Klausen, 2002). This move from observation-based studies to transcribed discourse allows the analyst to revisit and re-analyse material. It makes it possible to pick out the detailed patterns in actual interaction as opposed to the more broad-brush impressions that can be achieved from an observer's notes and reconstructions, and it allows other analysts to check and comment on the conclusions. The result is therefore an altogether more rigorous and defensible analysis from which to draw conclusions. For all these reasons, 'second wave' ethnography was the method of choice for this part of the study. What was also clear, as we examined studies of public deliberation, particularly the available case studies of citizens' juries, was that a second wave ethnography would represent a methodological advance on what had gone before. There is a further important point. If, as Wenger (1999) suggests, people in a new community of practice over time develop and share ways of talking and being together, then the only way to capture this with any accuracy is to have access to transcribed discourse in the ways we have suggested.

The film crew were highly skilled at filming unobtrusively and developed good working relations with participants. Citizens Council members reported that they had found the presence of the camera crew only noticeable in the initial stages of filming, thereafter becoming accustomed to them. This resonates with the results of other studies and with the good level of cooperation with the evaluation as a whole. Filming what was to become a changing format for council sessions occasionally caused problems. For instance, the researchers were not involved in the choice of venues for the meetings. In the first Council meeting the venue did not have separate rooms for small group work. Therefore, the recording of this was difficult and meant that it was hard for the transcribers to distinguish between groups, and equally hard to decipher who was speaking at any moment in time. Furthermore, the facilitators often changed the programme. These changes reflected the way that the Citizens Council meetings were developing, but it made the recording of sessions difficult at times, with the camera crew having to respond quickly to the changes. Nonetheless, these problems were relatively minor and, in all, 64 hours of recorded data were collected, including the bulk of the small group work and all the main sessions of the Council.

The recordings were transcribed following a detailed schema to create a verbatim record. Once the whole data corpus had been transcribed for each meeting, the transcripts were then checked against the video-recordings to ensure that they were as accurate as possible. The transcription was at a relatively gross level rather than fine-grain as was appropriate for the research questions. Overlaps, interruptions, pauses and other interactional features were thus not included in the transcription record. The transcribed data was also supplemented by the traditional method of using observation diaries. Observational notes of the fourth meeting were used, as planned, to give a check on the emerging analysis of the first three meetings. Details of the quantitative and qualitative procedures that were used are given in the chapters of Part II.

Studying the organisational context

Our initial theoretical frame stressed the always less than straightforward process of policy implementation (Hogwood and Gunn, 1984), and the importance of a sound understanding of the provenance of any policy development (Davies, 2000). We noted suggestions in the health policy literature that rhetoric had tended to outrun practice in the field of public involvement, and highlighted the likely challenge of making an effective 'join' between the results emerging from the Council and the mainstream activity of the organisation. We therefore set out to provide an account of the emergence of the Citizens Council, its initial shaping and its subsequent development, paying attention to the amendments and policy developments in the light of experience over the study period.

The design as originally specified consisted of three main elements: documentary analysis and review, including desk research of cognate areas; semi-structured face-to-face interviews with key players inside and outside the organisation; and ongoing monitoring of the responses to the work of the Council. All the formal interviews were recorded on audiotape to supplement the evaluators' interview and field notes.

The Institute's way of working stressed ongoing development, and the regular meetings of the Citizens Council steering committee in NICE were an important focus for this. We therefore observed the steering committee and relevant board meetings throughout the duration of the project, conducting further interviews with key players, including Vision 21, and holding liaison meetings with the project manager.

As the study progressed, agreements were negotiated to extend the initial design to reflect developments more fully. Importantly, this enabled us to observe the Institute's attempts to solve the problem of how to integrate the results of the Council members' deliberations into the existing work of the Board, the appraisals and guidelines programmes and their advisory committees. Thus in practice the data-gathering stage covered further formal and informal interviews, and an observational study of the meetings of the steering committee and the Board. In the event the work extended even further to cover the four so-called 'impact' workshops with members of the various advisory committees in the final weeks of the study period (see Chapter Seven). The result, while still working within constraints, was to move the design towards more of a total ethnography.

Preliminary scoping sessions were completed with the project manager, the executive director for resources and planning, and the clinical director. Documentary analysis and review followed, covering published corporate material, minutes of past Council steering committee meetings and press cuttings. Throughout the study further documentation was amassed, including corporate and business plans as they became available, lists of appraisals and guidelines programme activities, Board meeting minutes and documentation, and minutes of the Citizens Council steering committee before, during and after each of their (on average six-weekly) meetings. The Institute's website also furnished a wealth of information – one of the advantages of the organisation's commitment to transparency. (A listing of the documentation consulted can be found in Appendix 5.)

A total of 24 semi-structured face-to-face interviews was completed, the majority in the first six months of the project. Relationships forged early on with respondents bore fruit subsequently in informal opportunistic conversations before and after Board and committee meetings, during Council meetings, in telephone calls to confirm arrangements or ask for documentation, and in the parliamentary reception held for the Council members in October 2003. For a few respondents, additional formal interviews were also conducted later in the evaluation period, particularly towards the very end when the four implementation workshops with the appraisals and guidelines programme staff and committee members were observed. In addition, relevant staff from Vision 21, the arm's length agency handling Council member recruitment and meeting facilitation, were also interviewed. Since the recruitment and selection of Council members had already been conducted before the research started, we had to rely on existing documentation together with retrospective accounts. We visited Vision 21's offices in Manchester to inspect their database and procedures, and interview the staff involved. The second visit consisted entirely of a single in-depth interview with one of the directors of Vision 21, who gave as thorough an account of the process as commercial secrecy permitted. We needed to be sensitive to their concern for safeguarding information that gave them, as a business concern, commercial advantage. Such concerns, of course, are not always congruent with the needs of a research project.

Minutes and papers from committee meetings and interviews with the project manager also provided data for this part of the study.

In the early interviews particular attention was paid to the process of initial agenda setting. Accounts of the emergence of topics for the Council and how the Council's outputs might be used by and incorporated within the organisation were gathered. At NICE's request, a very early interim report was drawn up in January 2003 which included a short paper on the heterogeneous 'hopes, fears and suggestions' for the Citizens Council initiative from within NICE itself, enabling the organisation to access the views of its own (anonymised) members.

Subsequently detailed observation notes were completed for 11 meetings of the steering committee and six meetings of the board, as well as for two topic-setting meetings and one debriefing meeting between the steering committee and Vision 21. The four meetings of the Citizens Council and the two induction events for new Council members were also observed from the point of view of this part of the study, as was a parliamentary reception where the staff of NICE and the Council members and their families met socially. In particular, four workshops were organised by the project manager (two for the appraisals programme and two for the guidelines programme) to introduce the work of the Council to the staff of these programmes and the members of the committees in June and July 2004. Observations of these had not been planned, but formed the final, very late-in-the-day, but extremely informative, data gathering.

Studying the perceptions of Citizens Council members

Our research design proposed the use of diverse sources of information in order to understand the motivations for coming forward and changes in members' perceptions over time. This part of the study was conducted by the (then) College of Health. Helen Sheldon, an experienced researcher with the College, was responsible for this part of the research. We have been able to draw on her work for many of the quotes from individual citizens in the text, as well as from their written responses on Visions 21's feedback sheets. These have been used to add context and colour to the narrative.

A first round of semi-structured baseline telephone interviews was conducted with all 30 Council members before the first meeting of the Council, using an interview schedule designed to gather qualitative open-ended responses. These were tape-recorded, transcribed, and subjected to content analysis using NUDIST Vivo software and Framework Analysis (Ritchie and Spencer, 1994). Severe time constraints limited the choice of possibilities at this stage. The appointment of the research team was confirmed briefly before the induction meeting, leaving a period of around two weeks to contact a geographically dispersed group of 30 before the first Council meeting. Having secured the formal consent of Council members to the data collection at the induction event, these baseline telephone interviews took place in this brief period.

A second full round of one-to-one interviews, with each of the consenting Council members, was conducted following the third Council meeting. Conducting the interviews face-to-face in members' own homes or in a neutral venue of their choosing was strongly preferred as undoubtedly generative of the best quality data. However, circumstances again conspired to mean that telephone interviews were the only option. Additional information came from informal discussions at each of the Council meetings between Council members and members of the research team. We were also granted access to Vision 21's feedback sheets for each meeting. Material from these sources is interwoven through the account in this book. The final report on the project contains a chapter bringing all these sources together.

Citizens Council members cooperated well with the study. Despite their understandable early anxieties, they often came to seek us out at meetings, using us for informal discussions about how the meeting was going. Response rates to all aspects of the study proved to be high. A total of 28 telephone interviews (out of a possible 30) were completed in November 2002. Verbatim transcripts were checked with respondents. One person did not return the transcript and despite all efforts could not be contacted, so this transcript was not included in the analysis. As planned, the transcripts ($n=27$) were analysed using NUDIST Vivo, revisions requested by respondents being included in different fonts to indicate the status of the changed material. Two researchers coded each transcript into broad categories generated from the objectives identified for this part of the study. A detailed thematic analysis was then prepared, which formed one of the interim reports of the evaluation.

The second round of telephone interviews was conducted after the third Council meeting in December 2003. Out of a possible 30 interviews, 28 proved possible; one member was not present at the third meeting and another proved uncontactable. The interviews explored the way in which members' views of their role had changed, how they had experienced detailed aspects of the three meetings, and the lessons they had learned from all that had happened. As with the first round, interviews were recorded, transcribed, analysed and sent to respondents for checking. An interim progress report drawn from this data focused particularly on the ways in which views about the Council had changed. Subsequently it also proved possible to re-interrogate this dataset in order to develop insights into deliberation that linked directly to the observations of the Council in session.

Further details on the initial design as a species of 'third wave' evaluation and on the way in which it was modified and developed can be found in the final report on the project (see above).

Members of the Citizens Council, 2002-05

Vision 21, on NICE's behalf, recruited members of the public to be involved in the Citizens Council. The members of the council are listed below (this information is taken from the NICE website, www.nice.org.uk).

Citizens Council members for meetings one, two and three

- John Baldwin, an electrician who lives in Widnes, Cheshire.
- Auriol Britton, presently an unemployed aspiring writer who lives in Bristol, Avon.
- Brian Brown, an electrical engineer from Chester-le-Street, County Durham.
- Jennifer Brown, a clerical officer who lives in Derby, Derbyshire.
- Sylvia Brown, a retired local government officer who lives in London.
- Scott Chapman, a printer who lives in Corby, Northamptonshire.
- Tracey Christmas, an accountant who lives in Hull, East Yorkshire.
- Rod Crowshaw, a store assistant who lives in Castle Bromwich, West Midlands.
- Trevor Davison, a supervisor scaffolder who lives in Lincoln, Lincolnshire.
- Marie Goorun, a dressmaker and part-time French tutor who lives in Gillingham, Dorset.
- Mark Handley, a project manager who lives in Kingston-upon-Thames, Surrey.
- Susan Jones, a retail clerk who lives in Cardiff, Glamorgan.
- Rashad Khan, an administrator who lives in Keighley, West Yorkshire.
- Deborah Lee, a part-time advertisement make-up artist and housewife who lives in Bournemouth, Dorset.
- Raymond Longstaffe, a former builder who lives in Brecon, Powys.

- John MacGlashan, retired security officer, Liverpool, Merseyside.
- Melanie McClure, a mother of one who lives in Hebburn, Tyne and Wear.
- Susan McNeill, a secretary who lives in Market Harborough, Leicestershire.
- Anthony Messenger, an insurance broker who lives in Windsor, Berkshire.
- Sharon Morgan, a milliner who lives in Birmingham, West Midlands.
- Sunita Nanda, a local government officer, who lives in Middlesex.
- Bob Osborne, a retired former pilot who lives in Horsham, West Sussex.
- Paul Pendlebury, an assembly worker who lives in Preston, Lancashire.
- Audrey Pestell, a retired head teacher who lives in Woodhall Spa, Lincolnshire.
- Marie Raynor, a housewife who lives in Sale, Greater Manchester.
- Ian Simons, a taxi driver who lives in London.
- Colin Stewart, a self-employed IT systems advisor who lives in London.
- Fiona Taylor, a wine marketing assistant who lives in Sidbury, Devon.
- Peter Thomas, a teacher who lives in Rhondda, Cynon Taff.
- Judith Ward, a wood turner who lives near Stoke on Trent, Staffordshire.

The NICE website also provides the table below which gives details of statistics of the council make-up.

Demographics of the Citizens Council (meetings one, two and three)

Population (England and Wales) (%)	Criteria	Panel numbers required to match population statistics	Actual panel members meeting the criteria
10	under 25 years	3	4
20	over 60 years	6	6
12	disability	3	3
5 (10)	ethnic minority	3	4
13	home, student, unemployed	4	5
19	partly skilled/unskilled	6	4
25	skilled manual	7	8
26	skilled non-manual	8	7
14	managerial and technical	4	4
3	professional	1	3
49	male	15	15
51	female	15	15
95	live in England	28	27
5	live in Wales	2	3
7.9	East Midlands	2	2
10.2	East	3	3
4.8	North East	1	2
13.0	North West	4	4
15.2	South East	5	4
9.3	South West	3	4
10.0	West Midlands	3	3
9.5	Yorks & Humber	3	2
15.0	London	4	3

Source: www.nice.org.uk

Citizens Council members for meeting four

The intention was always that the Council would be periodically 'refreshed'. Ten names were selected randomly and replacements were found from the database held by Vision 21, to produce the following list of members for the fourth meeting.

- John Baldwin, an electrician who lives in Widnes, Cheshire.
- Auriol Britton, a singer working towards a diploma, who lives in Bristol, Avon.
- Brian Brown, an electrical engineer from Chester-le-Street, County Durham.
- Jennifer Brown, a clerical officer who lives in Derby, Derbyshire.
- Sylvia Brown, a retired local government officer who lives in London.

- Rod Crowshaw, a store assistant who lives in Castle Bromwich, West Midlands.
- Trevor Davison, a supervisor scaffolder who lives in Lincoln, Lincolnshire.
- Geraldine Fost, a retired careers guidance manager who lives in Hungerford, Berkshire.
- Lorna Girling, a part-time philosophy student and a housewife and mother of one who lives in Norfolk.
- Susan Glendinning (nee Jones), a part-time actress and clerical assistant who lives in Cardiff, Glamorgan.
- Marie Goorun, a dressmaker and part-time French tutor who lives in Gillingham, Dorset.
- Terry Hamer works on the cruise ships at the terminal in Southampton.
- Mark Handley, a project manager who lives in Kingston-upon-Thames, Surrey.
- Robert Jones, who works as a warehouse operative and is a football referee in his spare time and lives in Cwnbran, Wales.
- Arun Jotangia currently works for Manchester Airport and lives in Bolton.
- Rashad Khan, an administrator who lives in Keighley, West Yorkshire.
- John Mahoney, a former foreign editor for the BBC and for ITN News at Ten who lives in London.
- Melanie McClure, a mother of one who lives in Hebburn, Tyne and Wear.
- Susan McNeill, a secretary who lives in Market Harborough, Leicestershire.
- Anthony Messenger, an insurance broker who lives in Windsor, Berkshire.
- Sharon Morgan, a milliner who lives in Birmingham, West Midlands.
- Linda Moss, currently unemployed, trained as a TEFL teacher and now lives in Todmorden, West Yorkshire.
- Bob Osborne, a retired former pilot who lives in Horsham, West Sussex.
- Paul Pendlebury, an assembly worker who lives in Preston, Lancashire.
- Lisa Pompeo, a communications operator for the police who lives in Bradford.
- Helen Sabir worked for a while in human resources, and has recently moved to Huddersfield, where she is looking for suitable work.
- Ian Simons, a taxi driver who lives in London.

- Paddy Storrie, a secondary school headteacher who lives in Harpenden, Hertfordshire.
- Fiona Taylor, a wine marketing assistant who lives in Sidbury, Devon.
- Peter Thomas, a teacher who lives in Rhondda, Cynon Taff.
- Judith Ward, a wood turner who lives near Stoke on Trent, Staffordshire.

The NICE website also provides the table below which gives details of statistics of the council make-up.

Demographics of the Citizens Council (meeting four)

Population (England and Wales) (%)	Criteria	Panel numbers required to match population statistics	Actual panel members meeting the criteria
10	under 25 years	3	4
20	over 60 years	6	6
12	disability	3 or 4	3
5 (10)	ethnic minority	3	4
13	home, student, unemployed	4	5
19	partly skilled/unskilled	6	4
25	skilled manual	7	8
26	skilled non-manual	8	7
14	managerial and technical	4	4
3	professional	1	3
49	male	15	15
51	female	15	15
95	live in England	28	27
5	live in Wales	2	3
7.9	East Midlands	2	1
10.2	East	3	3
4.8	North East	1	2
13.0	North West	4	4
15.2	South East	2	4
9.3	South West	3	4
10.0	West Midlands	3	3
9.5	Yorks & Humber	3	2
15.0	London	4	3

Source: www.nice.org.uk

Detailed agenda for the four Citizens Council meetings

Meeting one (clinical need)

Thursday	Friday	Saturday
Introduction to the meeting from Mike Rawlins (NICE)	Citizens councillor members had a private session to discuss difficulties they were experiencing	A session with Helen from the evaluation team who explained the member study
Questions to Mike	Feedback to Vision 21	Questions to Helen
The council broke into three groups of 10 and prepared questions for the witnesses	Small group work using case studies to discuss what should be taken into account when deciding about clinical need with reference to: a) features of conditions b) features of patients c) weight the Institution gives to the various stakeholders	Witness presentation – Gavin McGreggor (North of England Manager for Carers UK) Questions to Gavin
Witness presentation – Chris Spry (Chair of OD Partnerships and former NHS chief executive)	Plenary session – each small group reported back on their discussions of the case studies	Witness presentation – Nigel Hughes (Chief Executive of the British Liver Trust)
Questions to Chris		Questions to Nigel

Meeting one (clinical need) contd.../

Thursday	Friday	Saturday
Witness presentation – Jackie Pollock (Patient representative) Questions to Jackie Pollock	A session with Margie from the evaluation team who explained the ethnographic study Questions to the evaluation team	The facilitators led a session about what the structure of the report would look like
Witness presentation – Richard Tiner (Medical Director of the Association of British Pharmaceutical Industries) Questions to Richard	Witness presentation – Bill Fulford (Psychiatrist and Philosopher) Questions to Bill	Small group work – worked on key points for the report
Witness presentation – Hugh Reeve (Medical Director of Clinical Governance at Morecombe Bay Primary Care Trust and part-time GP) Questions to Hugh	Witness presentation – Ruth McDonald (Research Fellow, Department for Applied Social Sciences, Manchester University and former NHS Finance Director) Questions to Ruth	Plenary review session – worked towards recommendations for the report
Plenary review session – Council recorded key points from witnesses' sessions	Witness presentation – Stephanie Sulliaman (Wandsworth Primary Care Trust, Nurse Specialist in Sickle Cell Anaemia) Questions to Stephanie	One Citizens Council member reported back to Andrew Dillon (NICE) about how the Citizens councillors found the first meeting
	Witness presentation – NICE panel – Carole Longson, Gillian Laing and Tom Dent Questions to NICE panel	Andrew Dillon thanked them for their efforts
	Plenary review session – Council recorded and discussed key points from witnesses	

Meeting two (age)

Wednesday evening	Thursday	Friday	Saturday
Feedback session from the evaluation team Questions to the evaluation team Two Citizens Council members reported back from the first report Andrew Dillon (NICE) welcomed the Citizens Council members to the meeting Questions to Andrew Ela Pathak-Sen (NICE) – session on ground rules	Introduction to the topic from Mike Rawlins (NICE) Questions to Mike	The council broke into four groups and worked on a role-play about how to distribute a grant allocation from a local health board that had money to spend on new treatments. They worked in role as four sub-committees of the board and had to prepare arguments for their case to be awarded the money	Witness presentation – Mark Drayton (Consultant Neontologist at University Hospital of Wales) Questions to Mark
	The council broke into three groups of 10 and prepared questions for the witnesses	Plenary session where each small group presented their cases followed by a debate about which group should be awarded the money Plenary session where the group reviewed the debate	Citizens Council members wrote down in twos how they would answer the question
	Plenary session – discussed initial thoughts on the question	Witness presentation – John Grimley Evans (Professor of Clinical Gerontology, Nuffield Department of Clinical Medicine) Questions to John	The council worked in small groups on recommendations for the report

Meeting two (age) contd.../

Wednesday evening	Thursday	Friday	Saturday
	Witness presentation – NICE panel Questions to NICE panel	Witness presentation – Karen Newbigging (Director of the Centre for Mental Health Services Development England) Questions to Karen	Plenary review session – reported back from small groups Made recommendations for the report
	Witness presentation – Harry Cayton (Chief Executive of the Alzheimer's Society, Director of Patient Experience and Public Involvement, Department of Health) Questions to Harry	Witness presentation – Chris Heneghan (Council of the Royal College of Anaesthetists, Specialist in Intensive Care at the Nevill Hall Hospital, Abergavenny) Questions to Chris	Ray Luff (Non-Executive Director of NICE, board member of the Public Health Laboratory Service) thanked the Citizens Council
	Witness presentation – Alan Williams (Professor of Economics, Centre for Health Economics, University of York) Questions to Alan	NEXUS discussed press coverage	
	The council broke into three groups of 10 to prepare and worked on case studies about age-related conditions in order to demonstrate the decision-making process that NICE face	Plenary review session – Council recorded and discussed key points from witnesses	
	Plenary review session – Council recorded and discussed key points from witnesses		

Meeting three (age)

Thursday	Friday	Saturday
Introduction to the third meeting and discussion of the retirement policy and the new activities that have been included into the meeting (eg use of camcorder and tape recorder to record views and exercise involving pictures and money)	Witness presentation – David Barnett (Chair of NICE's Appraisal Committee) Carole Longson (NICE) Questions to David and Carole	The council worked in small groups on recommendations for the report
Plenary group session with a 'lucky dip' exercise around moral dilemmas	David and Carole led two groups through a mock appraisal committee	Mike Rawlins (NICE) session with the Citizens Council
Introduction to the question from Mike Rawlins and Andrew Dillon (NICE) Questions to Mike and Andrew	Witness presentation – David Barnett (Chair of NICE's Appraisal Committee) Questions to David	Plenary session where Citizens councillors wrote individual recommendations for the report and discussed these as a group
Witness presentation – Paul Dolan (Health Economist) Questions to Paul	David and Carole led two groups through a mock appraisal committee	Discussion of future meetings and close of meeting
Witness presentation – NCB presented the views of young people Questions to NCB	Plenary session – reviewed in threes a) what are main strengths/weaknesses of appraisal process b) what had learned to help answer the question	
Plenary review session – worked in threes to isolate age and take into account whether treatment is cost-effective or not	Witness presentation – Ray Tallis (Professor) Questions to Ray	
	The council worked in small groups on aspects of the question	
	Plenary review session – worked on the rationale behind their answers to the question	

Meeting four (confidential enquiries)

Thursday	Friday	Saturday
Introduction and welcome session with the 10 new members Reminder of ground rules Plenary session on initial thoughts on the topic	Witness presentations – staff from Brighton and Sussex University hospitals: Julia Budnik (Senior Clinical Effectiveness Facilitator), Sarah Danko (Clinical Effectiveness and Audit Manager) and Charles Turton (Medical Director)	Witness presentation – Arnold Simanowitz (Partner in the solicitors' firm Simanowitz & Brown until 1981, then Chief Executive of the charity Action for Victims of Medical Accidents) Questions to Arnold
Witness panel presentation – Christabel Hargraves (Chief Executive of the National Confidential Enquiry into Patient Outcome and Death) Questions Richard Congdon (Chief Executive CEMACH) Questions to panel	Worked in small groups with above staff from Brighton and Sussex University hospitals – discussed what issues they wanted to Swapped speakers and groups	Plenary session where Citizens councillors wrote individual recommendations for the report and then discussed these in groups
Witness panel presentation – Kirsten Windfurh (Project Manager, Centre for Suicide Prevention 2002, Senior Project Manager for the National Confidential Inquiry into Suicide and Homicide, 2003) Nav Kapoor (Assistant Director, Senior Lecturer in Psychiatry) Questions to the panel	Plenary session which discussed the big issues – individual Council members offered the chance to choose an issue and form a group – Council members then moved between groups and discussed issues	Closing review session

Meeting four (confidential enquiries) contd.../

Thursday	Friday	Saturday
Witness panel presentation – Louise Parker (NICE R&D), Chris Hargraves (Chief Executive NCEPOD) and Richard Congdon (Chief Executive, CEMACH) present the case for exemption for individual consent. Questions to panel	Witness panel presentation – Hannah Godfrey (Junior Barrister of Lincoln's Inn) and Richard Congdon (Chief Executive, CEMACH) Questions to panel	Evaluation team thank the Citizens Council members
Questionnaire handed out on the questions for Council members to complete	The Council worked in small groups preparing to debate the opposing sides represented by Hannah and Richard	Mike Rawlins (NICE)
Witness panel presentation – Sean Kirwan (Digital Policy Development Officer at the Department of Health and Secretary of the Patient Information Advisory Group) Karen Thompson (User Involvement Manager at Diabetes UK) Questions to the panel	Debate – Hannah and Richard summarise then open up debate Vote	Ela Pathak thanked the Citizens Council members
Citizens Council members asked to swap places with person next to them	Reflection time	

Meeting four (confidential enquiries) contd.../

Thursday	Friday	Saturday
Mike Rawlins (NICE) and Andrew Dillon fed back thoughts on the age report and discussed how NICE were implementing the decisions/impact of the Citizens Council Also introduce the topic		
The Council work in groups of four to discuss whether the national confidential enquiries should be requested to seek prior informed consent about whose identifiable data is used in research		
Plenary review session where small groups reported back their discussions		

National Institute for Clinical Excellence: background and developments

The National Institute for Clinical Excellence (NICE) is one of the new government arm's length agencies, and although its history to date is not long, it has been eventful. As an organisation it presents researchers with significant challenges due to its ever-evolving nature. What can be said of its organisational structure and functioning at one moment does not necessarily hold true the next. Consequently we shall here describe NICE first as it was at the time of our data gathering, and then as it is at the time of writing this book.

At the time of our research

The Institute was established as a Special Health Authority and part of the NHS in April 2000, to promote clinical excellence and the effective use of resources in England and Wales. As one of a series of new regulatory bodies, it had arisen in the context of government moves designed to set clear national standards and improve the quality of care in Britain's NHS. Its task was to bring together and review evidence for clinical practice, making recommendations both as to the clinical effectiveness and the cost-effectiveness of particular interventions (DH, 1997). The aim was that healthcare should become more responsive to individual need, more effective in drawing on the best available clinical evidence, and also more economically efficient (DH,1998: para 2.3). Institute assessments should include "impact on quality of life, relief of pain or disability" (NICE, 2000: Annex C: para 10), as well as having regard for the clinical priorities of the NHS.

At the time of this study (2002-04) NICE was engaged in producing guidance in three areas of health:

- the use of new and existing medicines and treatments within the NHS – technology appraisals;

- the appropriate treatment and care of people with specific diseases and conditions within the NHS in England and Wales – clinical guidelines;
- whether interventional procedures used for diagnosis or treatment are safe enough and work well enough for routine use – interventional procedures.

The appraisals programme was supported by three appraisals committees. The guidelines programme was supported by guideline review groups and guideline development groups drawn from seven national collaborating centres. And the interventional procedures programme was also supported by an advisory committee.

In the first five years of the Institute's life, appraisals work was the most prominent activity. Advice to the NHS covered a range of drugs, for example, Relenza for 'flu and Taxanes for breast cancer. NICE also formulated pronouncements on medical devices, for example, on asthma inhalers and implantable cardioverter defibrillators. Its guidance in all cases takes the form of a reasoned assessment of whether an intervention can be deemed a clinically effective and cost-effective use of NHS resources, indicating appropriateness in general or for particular subgroups, or recommending, for example, a period of further clinical trial. Documents are distributed widely in the NHS, are available on the Institute's website and are also intended for and in some cases used by patients and the public. The outputs of the Institute are termed 'authoritative guidance' and clinical discretion in relation to individual patients is acknowledged in the documentation setting up the Institute and in its publications.

The detailed work programme of the Institute is a matter for the Department of Health and Welsh Assembly. NICE itself, however, consults widely on this and makes suggestions.

In terms of overall structure, NICE employed a core staff of 92, and received annual funding of just under £18 million (August 2004). The board of the Institute comprised eight non-executive directors (including the chair and vice-chair) and four executive directors (including the chief executive). The Partners Council provides a forum for the exchange of ideas, and has a statutory duty to meet annually to review the Institute's Annual Report. Members include patients and representatives of patient-focused organisations, professional organisations and relevant healthcare industries. Patient involvement is an important feature for NICE and in-house resources have increasingly been added to support this. A new

Patient, Carer and Public Involvement Programme was announced in January 2005 to those involved in producing NICE guidance. The document added that the Citizens Council continues to bring "the views of the public to NICE decision-making" (www.nice.org.uk, accessed 4 November 2005).

At the time of writing

Shortly after the completion of this study, on 1 April 2005, NICE incorporated the former Health Development Agency, becoming the National Institute for Health and Clinical Excellence. The new organisation issued for consultation a new operating model for the new 'shape' of the Institute:

> NICE is the independent organisation responsible for providing national guidance on the promotion of good health and the prevention and treatment of ill health. On 1 April 2005 NICE joined with the Health Development Agency to become the new National Institute for Health and Clinical Excellence (also to be known as NICE).... The National Institute for Health and Clinical Excellence will produce guidance in three areas of health:
>
> - Public health – guidance on the promotion of good health and the prevention of ill health for those working in the NHS, local authorities and the wider public and voluntary sector
> - Health technologies – guidance on the use of new and existing medicines, treatments and procedures within the NHS
> - Clinical practice – guidance on the appropriate treatment and care of people with specific diseases and conditions within the NHS. (www.nice.org.uk, accessed 3 August 2005)

The intention was that guidance would now be produced by three centres within NICE: the Centre for Public Health Excellence, the Centre for Health Technology Evaluation and the Centre for Clinical Practice.

Up-to-date and historical information is available on NICE's website (www.nice.org.uk). This includes details of and reports from the Citizens Council. For some independent academic commentary on the Institute, see, for example, Appleby and Coote (2002); Ham and Robert (2003), and an early collection of critical essays under a medical imprint (Miles et al, 2000).

Key data sources

This appendix lists major documentary sources, published and unpublished, from NICE and from Vision 21, as used in the course of the study.

NICE

Printed publications

Corporate publications

'Annual Report 2001/2002 and summary financial statement' (September 2002)
'Annual Report 2002/2003 and summary financial statement'/ 'Addroddiad Blynyddol 2002/2003 a chrynodeb o'r adroddiad ariannol' (September 2003)
'Board meeting: agenda and papers' (18 September 2002)
'Board meeting: agenda and papers' (15 January 2003)
'Board meeting: agenda and papers' (19 March 2003)
'Board meeting: agenda and papers' (16 July 2003)
'Board meeting: agenda and papers' (21 January 2004)
'Board meeting: agenda and papers' (17 March 2004)
'Board meeting: agenda and papers' (21 July 2004)
'Business plan 2002-03' (September 2002)
'Business plan 2003-04' (September 2003)
'Corporate plan 2002-05' (September 2002)
'Corporate plan 2003-06' (September 2003)

Information, guides, etc

'A guide to NICE' (CD-ROM, December 2002; pamphlet March 2003; pamphlet April 2004)
'A guide to our work'/'Cannlaw I'n Gwaith' (nd [November 1999])
'Guidance for patient/carer groups', Technology Appraisals Process Series No 3 (June 2001)

'Guide to the technology appraisal process', Technology Appraisals Process Series No 1 (June 2001)

'Information for national collaborating centres and guideline development groups', The Guideline Development Process Series No 3 (December 2001)

'Information for stakeholders', The Guideline Development Process Series No 2 (December 2001)

'Information for the public and the NHS'/'Gwybodaeth i'r Cyhoedd ac i'r NHS', The Guideline Development Process Series No 1 (December 2001)

'National collaborating centres: developing clinical guidelines and audit advice for the NHS' (nd)

Examples of guidance publications

'Guidance for October 2003' (comprising Interventional Procedure Guidance 13-16, Clinical Guidelines 6-7, Technology Appraisals 69-71)

'Guidance for February 2004' (comprising Interventional Procedure Guidance 40-45, Clinical Guidelines 11-12)

'Guidance on home compared with hospital haemodialysis for patients with end-stage renal failure', Technology Appraisal Guidance No 48 (September 2002)

'Protocol-based care: underpinning improvement' (November 2002), joint publication with NHS Modernisation Agency

'Summary of guidance issued to the NHS in England and Wales' (issue 4, April 2002; issue 5, October 2002; issue 7, October 2003)

'Treating and managing schizophrenia (core interventions): understanding NICE' (December 2002)

Website publications

Information on Citizens Council

'A short introduction to the Citizens Council', www.nice.org.uk/article.asp?a=35543, accessed 23 October 2002

'Common questions and answers on the Citizens Council', www.nice.org.uk/article.asp?a=35546, accessed 23 October 2002

General information

'Common questions', www.nice.org.uk/cat.asp?c=129, accessed 27 September 2002

'Foreword', Frank Dobson, www.nice.org.uk/cat.asp?c=287, accessed 18 March 2003

'General information on the work of NICE', www.nice.org.uk/cat.asp?c=57703, accessed 23 September 2003

'Introduction', www.nice.org.uk/Embcat.asp?page=oldsite/back/policy/1stclass/1st_intro.htm, accessed 18 March 2003

'Secretary of State's Speech', Frank Dobson, www.nice.org.uk/Embcat.asp?page=oldsite/back/frank_dobson.htm&d=907, accessed 18 March 2003

'Setting quality standards', www.nice.org.uk/Embcat.asp?page=oldsite/back/policy/1stclass/1st_chp2.htm, accessed 18 March 2003

'Speech to St Paul International Health Care, Annual Lecture', www.nice.org.uk/article.asp?a=334, accessed 18 March 2003

'The National Institute for Clinical Excellence (NICE)', www.nice.org.uk/Embcat.asp?page=oldsite/back/policy/1stclass/1st_nice.htm, accessed 18 March 2003

'Welcome', Prof Sir Michael Rawlins, www.nice.org.uk/cat.asp?c=137, accessed 27 September 2002

Information on the Institute's organisation and work

'Achieving a patient and carer focus for the Institute's work' (December 1999), www.nice.org.uk/article.asp?a=453, accessed 8 April 2003

'Contact details for PIU staff', www.nice.org.uk/page.aspx?o=113704, accessed 23 May 2004

'Information about the Patient Involvement Unit', www.nice.org.uk/page.aspx?o=201780, accessed 23 May 2004

'Job vacancies: vacancies at NICE: associate guidelines director', www.nice.org.uk/cat.asp?c=80669, accessed 4 August 2003

'Job vacancies: vacancies at NCCs/PIU: half-time patient involvement project manager: national clinical guidelines', accessed 12 August 2003

'NICE Partners Council', www.nice.org.uk/article.asp?a=334, accessed 27 September 2002

'Patient Involvement Unit for NICE', www.nice.org.uk/page.aspx?o=73135, accessed 23 May 2004

'Questionnaires: pilot – do you want to suggest a topic for the NICE work programme?', www.nice.org.uk/article.asp?a=44901, accessed 23 December 2002

'Review of appraisals process and methodology', www.nice.org.uk/cat.asp?c=81933, accessed 5 August 2003

Press releases

2001/038 (22 November 2001) 'NICE to seek advice from new Citizens Council', www.nice.org.uk/article.asp?a=24940, accessed 28 November 2002

2002/044A (19 August 2002) 'UK's first Citizens Council being established by NICE'

2002/044B (nd) 'Have your say in health', www.nice.org.uk/article.asp?a=35552, accessed 29 August 2002

2002/048 (24 September 2002) 'Outstanding public response to join NICE's Citizens Council', www.nice.org.uk/article.asp?a=37058, accessed 28 November 2002

2002/049 (3 October 2002) 'Appointment of Professor Leon Fine as non-executive director of NICE', www.nice.org.uk/article.asp?a=37256, accessed 24 October 2002

2002/056 (8 November 2002) 'NICE announces members of first UK Citizens Council'

2002/057 (8 November 2002) 'Members of NICE Citizens Council react to appointment', www.nice.org.uk/article.asp?a=39077, accessed 8 November 2002

2002/061 (19 November 2002) 'First meeting of NICE Citizens Council will discuss clinical need', www.nice.org.uk/article.asp?a=40122, accessed 28 November 2002

2003/031 (17 July 2003) 'Research & Development programme established: Professor Sir Michael Marmot to chair R&D committee: two R&D associate directors appointed'

2003/03 (22 January 2003) 'Recommendations from Citizens Council on clinical need have immediate impact on NICE'

2003/034 (4 August 2003) 'Review of the appraisal process and methodology – NICE publishes consultation documents'

2003/035 (9 August 2003) 'Response to speculation on the NICE fertility guideline'

2003/055 (20 October 2003) 'Patient Involvement Unit transfers to the National Institute for Clinical Excellence'

2003/067 (nd) 'NICE consults on new strategy to strengthen guidance and improve quality of patient care'

2004/024 (13 May 2004) 'Groundbreaking work of NICE's Citizens Council continues as new members are welcomed'

2004/025 (20 May 2004) 'NICE launches programme of work to support implementation of its guidance in the NHS'

Other external communications

The Citizens Council

'Citizens Council: general texts (50-500 words)' (nd)

'Citizens Council: some common questions and answers' (August 2002)

'Cyngor Dinasyddion' (nd)

PowerPoint presentations (2) on Citizens Council (nd)

PowerPoint presentations (set of three): 'The Citizens Council' (nd), 'How were topics chosen for the Citizens Council?' by Peter Littlejohns (nd), 'How the Citizens Council deliberates by Vision 21' (nd)

Miscellaneous

E-newsletter (Nov 2002, Dec 2002, Jan 2003, Feb 2003, March 2003, June 2003, Oct 2003)

'Clinical excellence 2002: International Health Technology Assessment and Guidelines Conference: Annual Conference and Exhibition', conference programme and registration form (December 2002)

'NICE: opportunity or threat', Anne-Toni Rodgers, summary report to meeting of Chartered Institute of Marketing, Royal Counties Branch Health Care Group (January 2000)

'NICE – single line descriptors' (nd)

Internal documents

Committee papers

Citizens Council steering committee meetings (17 April 2002, 11 June 2002, 31 July 2002, 17 September 2002, 29 October 2002, 13 November 2002, 17 December 2002, 19 February 2003, 16 April 2003, 5 June 2003, 22 July 2003, 4 September 2003, 29 October 2003, 14 January 2004, 10 March 2004, 20 April 2004, 9 June 2004)

Topic setting meetings (16 July 2002, 24 January 2003, 11 March 2003)

Meetings with Vision 21 (10 September 2002, 5 June 2003)
Impact workshops (17 June 2004, 7 July 2004, 15 July 2004, 28 July 2004)

The Citizens Council

'Agency brief •Tender1: Recruitment of the Council members' (nd [June 2002])
'Agency brief •Tender2: Organising, facilitating and reporting on the Council meetings' (nd [June 2002])
'An introduction to the Citizens Council', NICE and Vision 21 (nd)
'Citizens Council draft, policy in confidence', Prof Sir Michael Rawlins, Chairman (October 2000)
'Citizens Council costs' (October 2004)
'Citizens Council operating model' (version 3, [3] April 2002; October 2002)
'Invitation to tender: evaluation of the NICE Citizens Council' (nd), www.nice.org.uk/Docref.asp?d=36590, accessed 28 November 2002
'Issues raised by certain aspects of the operating model', Citizens Council Project Manager (12 April 2002)
'National Institute for Clinical Excellence: Citizens Council', M.D. Rawlins (June 2002)
'NICE Citizens Council', Memo, From: Chris Ham, To: Liam Donaldson, Sarah Mullally, Andy McKeon; cc Simon Stevens, Michael Rawlins, Jo Lenaghan (27 February 2001)
'NICE Citizens Council chair's paper' (June 2002)
'Vision 21's proposal to recruit the National Institute for Clinical Excellence Citizens Council' (nd)
'Vision 21's proposal to organise, facilitate and report on the National Institute for Clinical Excellence Citizens Council' (nd)

Miscellaneous

'Framework document' (nd)
'Guide to the methods of technology appraisal', draft for consultation (August 2003)
'Guide to the technology appraisal process', draft for consultation (August 2003)
'Interim guide to the interventional procedures programme', version 1 (nd)
'NICE communication strategy' (26 July 2002)

'NICE management structure', diagram (nd [Sept 2003])

'NICE organogram' (nd)

'Planning and resources report: incorporating the finance report for the period 1 April to 30 September 2002' (20 November 2002)

'Research and development strategy: consultation document' (December 2003)

'Scientific and social value judgements', Michael D. Rawlins and Anthony J. Culler, draft (nd [September 2003])

'The guidelines development process: an overview', draft for consultation (July 2003)

Vision 21

Advertisement for councillors and list of placements

'Citizens' juries'

Evaluations of induction and first Council meeting from councillors' evaluation forms

'Hard-to-reach groups'

'How Vision 21 selected Citizens Council members'

'Listening and learning'

'Reaching the parts others can't reach', Greater Manchester CVO Information Bulletin (April 2002)

'Reputation audits'

Statistics on make-up of Citizens Council

'Tenants' views'

'Vision 21'

'Working with Vision 21'

Index